FIRST AID
FOR ANIMALS

FIRST AID
FOR ANIMALS

PIERO FORTUNATI

Illustrations by Cristina Girard

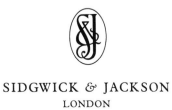

SIDGWICK & JACKSON
LONDON

Additional material by
Bruno Bassano (Wild Animals)
Marco Miglietti (Birds)
Cesare Pierbattisti (Small Mammals)

The publisher wishes to thank
Attilio Sosso for his assistance

Veterinary consultant: B.M. Bush, BVSc, PhD, FRCVS,
Royal Veterinary College, University of London

Photography: Lia Stein

First published in Great Britain in 1989 by
Sidgwick & Jackson Limited

ISBN 0–283–99903–9

Translated by Paul Foulkes
Additional material translated by John Gilbert

Filmset by Photospeed, London

Printed and bound in Italy by Arnoldo Mondadori Editore S.p.A., Verona
for Sidgwick & Jackson Limited
1 Tavistock Chambers, Bloomsbury Way
London WC1A 2SG

CONTENTS

INTRODUCTION

Anyone who owns a pet will know how easily animals can be the victims of accidents. In these situations your immediate intention is to give first aid to the animal in the best way you can and to ensure the rapid intervention of a vet. However, for many reasons it is often not possible for a vet to see the animal as soon as might be needed. In these cases a fuller awareness of possible injuries the animal may have sustained, and the immediate first-aid measures you can take, is of great value.

Giving first aid to an injured or sick animal is not always easy and, naturally, there is always the fear of worsening the situation. This book gives all the vital information and advice necessary to understand how you can treat an animal in an emergency in the simplest, safest and most effective way. It deals with a series of emergencies in which your initial intervention is both possible and useful. Each one is described and outlined clearly, many with detailed illustrations and instructions in steps, so you will be able to carry out the preliminary first aid confidently. Later it will be the vet who prescribes the correct drugs or appropriate treatment for the animal, but in the meantime you will at least be able to ensure the animal is kept safe and comfortable, with minimum threat to its health. Clearly, the information given in the book could never substitute the work of the veterinary surgeon. It should only serve to precede and complement subsequent veterinary treatment in a way that will make the recovery process more rapid and successful.

The book is divided into four parts. The first contains the basic principles of giving first aid to dogs, cats, small mammals and birds. The second and third parts concern the most frequent emergencies that will require first aid. The fourth part of the book outlines the various aspects of reproduction in dogs and cats and finally there is some basic information on how to recover stray animals and deal with injured wild animals.

FIRST AID
BASIC PRINCIPLES

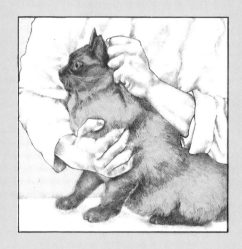

ANATOMICAL DIAGRAMS

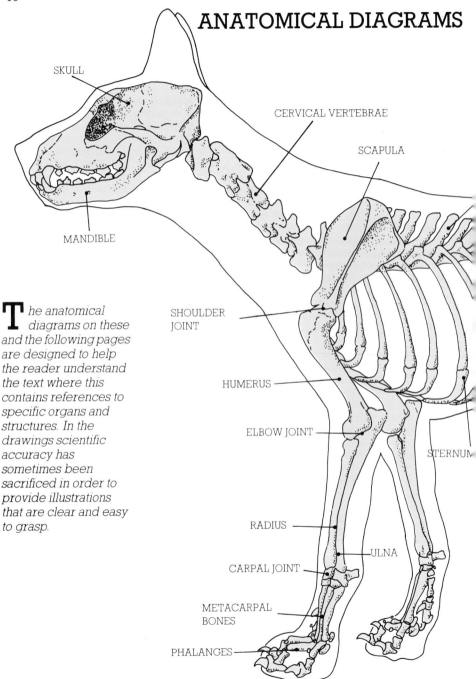

The anatomical diagrams on these and the following pages are designed to help the reader understand the text where this contains references to specific organs and structures. In the drawings scientific accuracy has sometimes been sacrificed in order to provide illustrations that are clear and easy to grasp.

SKULL

CERVICAL VERTEBRAE

SCAPULA

MANDIBLE

SHOULDER JOINT

HUMERUS

ELBOW JOINT

STERNUM

RADIUS

ULNA

CARPAL JOINT

METACARPAL BONES

PHALANGES

Skeleton of dog

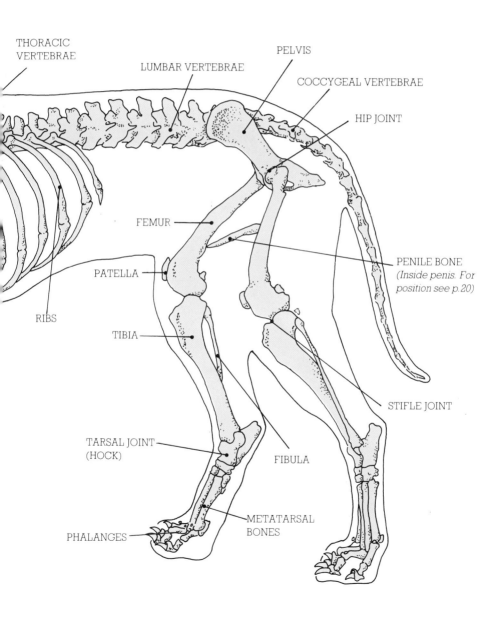

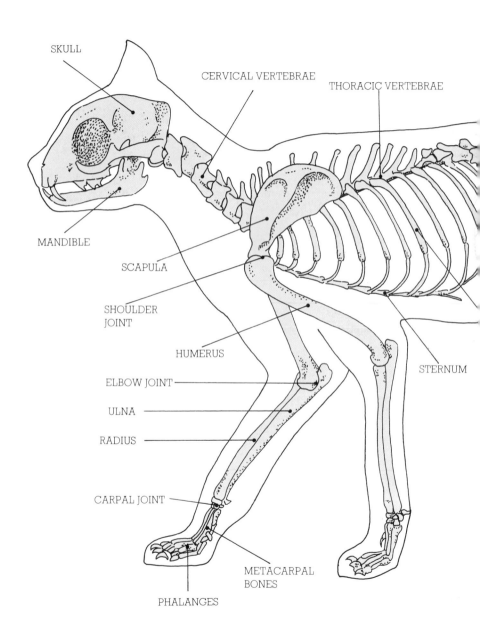

SKULL

CERVICAL VERTEBRAE

THORACIC VERTEBRAE

MANDIBLE

SCAPULA

SHOULDER
JOINT

HUMERUS

STERNUM

ELBOW JOINT

ULNA

RADIUS

CARPAL JOINT

METACARPAL
BONES

PHALANGES

Skeleton of cat

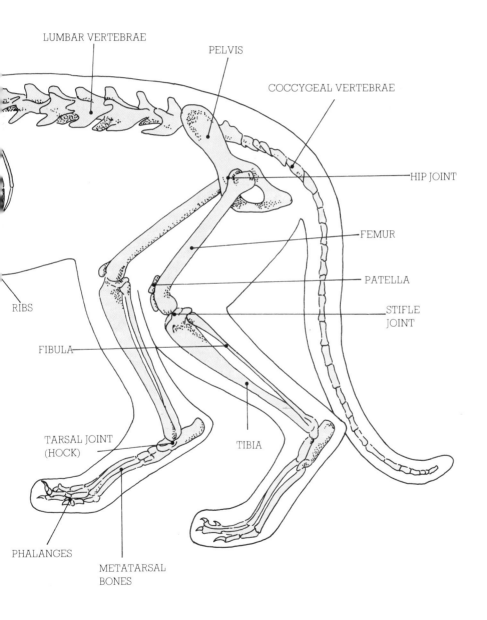

LUMBAR VERTEBRAE

PELVIS

COCCYGEAL VERTEBRAE

HIP JOINT

FEMUR

PATELLA

STIFLE JOINT

RIBS

FIBULA

TARSAL JOINT (HOCK)

TIBIA

PHALANGES

METATARSAL BONES

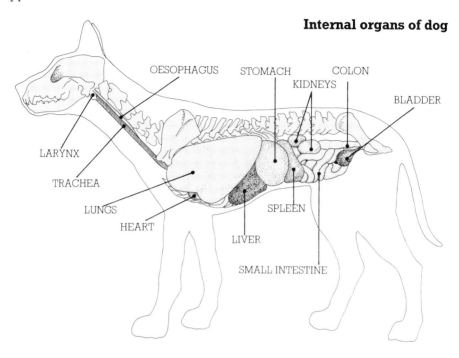

Internal organs of dog

OESOPHAGUS   STOMACH   COLON
KIDNEYS
BLADDER
LARYNX
TRACHEA
LUNGS   SPLEEN
HEART
LIVER
SMALL INTESTINE

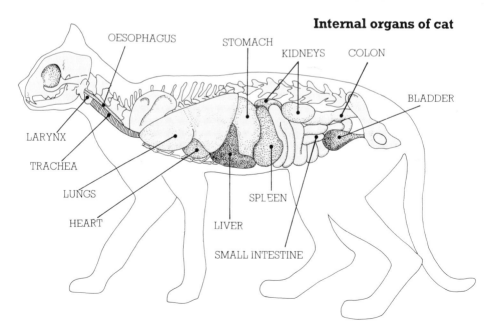

Internal organs of cat

OESOPHAGUS   STOMACH   COLON
KIDNEYS
BLADDER
LARYNX
TRACHEA
LUNGS   SPLEEN
HEART   LIVER
SMALL INTESTINE

Cross section of eye of dog and cat

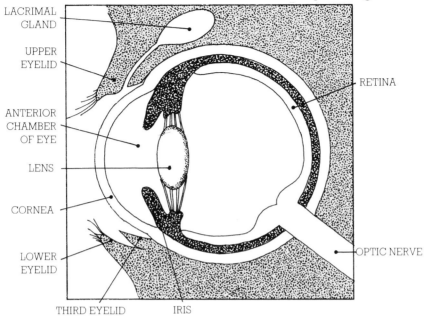

LACRIMAL
GLAND

UPPER
EYELID

ANTERIOR
CHAMBER
OF EYE

LENS

CORNEA

LOWER
EYELID

RETINA

OPTIC NERVE

THIRD EYELID   IRIS

Eye of cat   **Eye of dog**

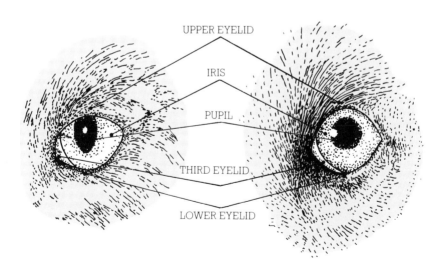

UPPER EYELID

IRIS

PUPIL

THIRD EYELID

LOWER EYELID

Cross section of ear

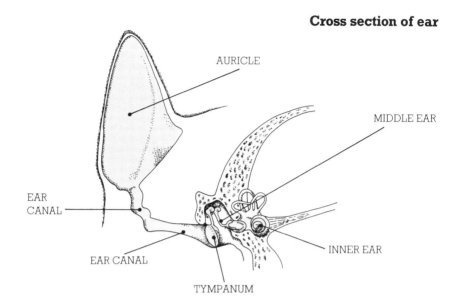

AURICLE

MIDDLE EAR

EAR
CANAL

INNER EAR

EAR CANAL

TYMPANUM

Ear of dog

Ear of cat

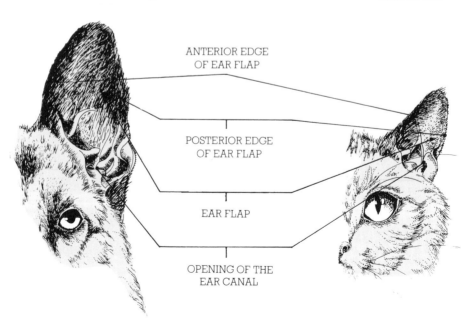

ANTERIOR EDGE
OF EAR FLAP

POSTERIOR EDGE
OF EAR FLAP

EAR FLAP

OPENING OF THE
EAR CANAL

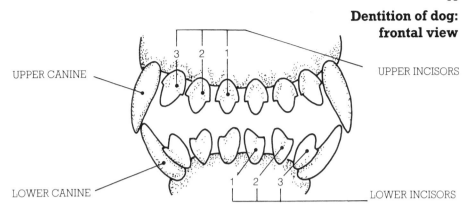

Dentition of dog: frontal view

UPPER CANINE

UPPER INCISORS

3 2 1

LOWER CANINE

LOWER INCISORS

1 2 3

Dentition of cat: frontal view

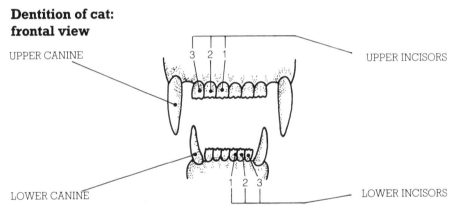

UPPER CANINE

UPPER INCISORS

3 2 1

LOWER CANINE

LOWER INCISORS

1 2 3

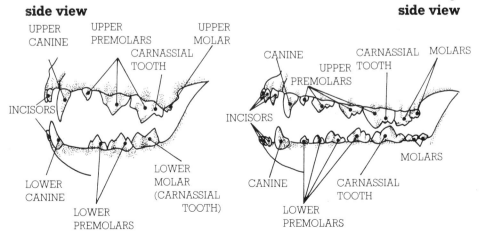

Dentition of adult cat: side view

UPPER CANINE

UPPER PREMOLARS

UPPER MOLAR

CARNASSIAL TOOTH

INCISORS

LOWER CANINE

LOWER PREMOLARS

LOWER MOLAR (CARNASSIAL TOOTH)

Dentition of adult dog: side view

CANINE

UPPER PREMOLARS

CARNASSIAL TOOTH

MOLARS

INCISORS

CANINE

LOWER PREMOLARS

CARNASSIAL TOOTH

MOLARS

Nose of dog

Nose of cat

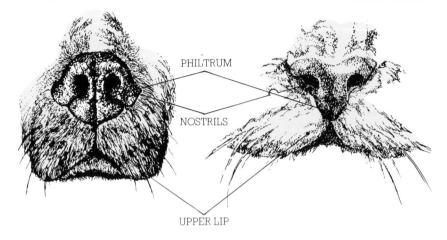

PHILTRUM

NOSTRILS

UPPER LIP

Cross section of skull and neck of dog

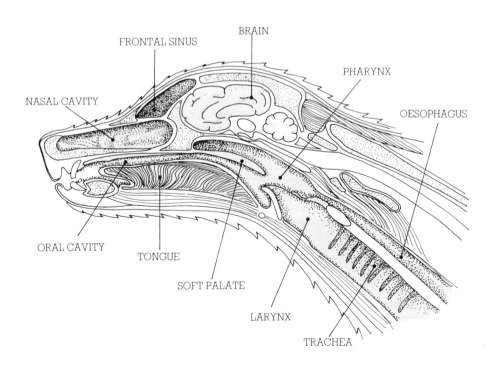

FRONTAL SINUS

BRAIN

PHARYNX

NASAL CAVITY

OESOPHAGUS

ORAL CAVITY

TONGUE

SOFT PALATE

LARYNX

TRACHEA

Cross section of skin and subcutaneous tissue

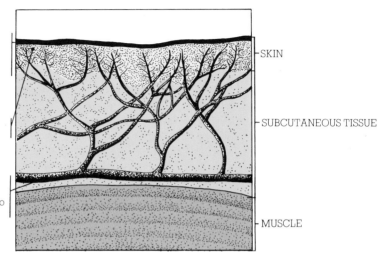

EPIDERMIS: the surface layer of skin, made up of layers of cells

DERMIS: the deeper, connective tissue layer of the skin

BLOOD VESSELS: run through the subcutaneous tissue and send branches to the skin

SKIN

SUBCUTANEOUS TISSUE

MUSCLE

Schematic drawing of a joint

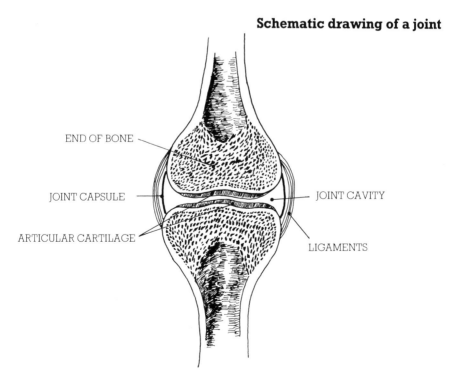

END OF BONE

JOINT CAPSULE

ARTICULAR CARTILAGE

JOINT CAVITY

LIGAMENTS

Genital apparatus of dog

Male

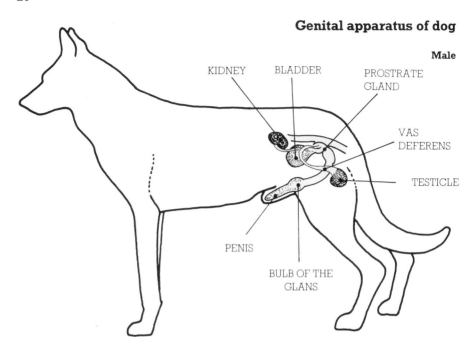

KIDNEY   BLADDER   PROSTRATE GLAND

VAS DEFERENS

TESTICLE

PENIS

BULB OF THE GLANS

Genital apparatus of dog

Female

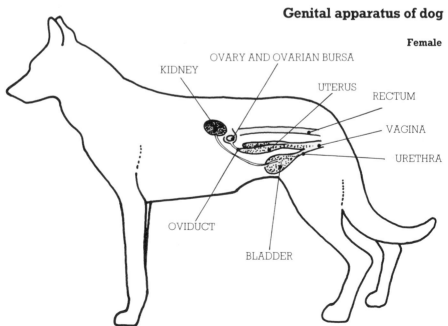

OVARY AND OVARIAN BURSA

KIDNEY

UTERUS   RECTUM

VAGINA

URETHRA

OVIDUCT

BLADDER

Genital apparatus of cat

Male

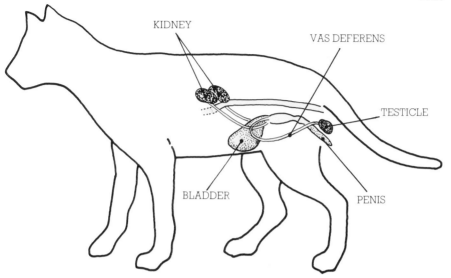

KIDNEY

VAS DEFERENS

TESTICLE

BLADDER

PENIS

Genital apparatus of cat

Female

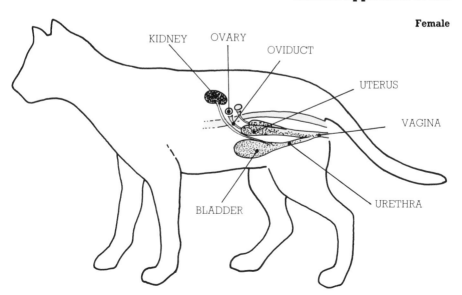

KIDNEY OVARY OVIDUCT

UTERUS

VAGINA

BLADDER

URETHRA

Skeleton and internal organs of rabbit

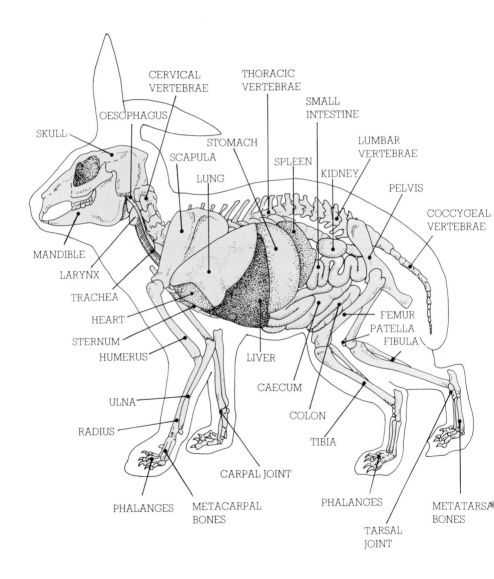

Skeleton and internal organs of birds

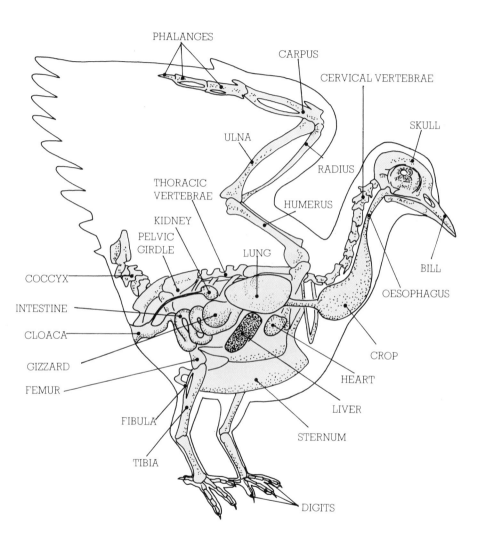

RESTRAINING

For first aid to be successful, the animal should ideally co-operate with you. Unfortunately it will often rebel and reject help, either from fear and pain or because of its temperament and lack of training. In such cases it must be restrained and forced to keep still, so that a helper will be protected and can act confidently without sudden movements worsening the situation. The animal must be held firmly but without violence; a strong, secure grip which is also reassuring is far more effective than a harsh, nervous one.

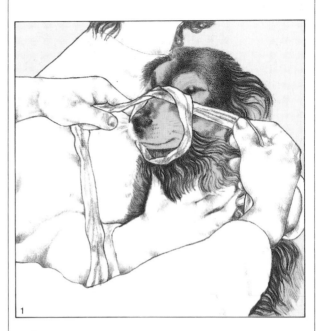

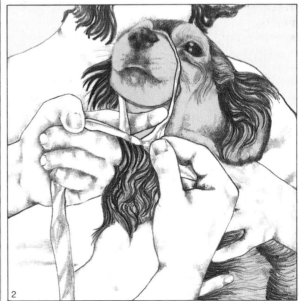

Dogs

■ **Restraining the mouth**

■ First you must assess whether the dog might bite you. This can easily be prevented by applying a muzzle or, if this is not available, by tying its jaws together with a soft strap or length of wide tape.

– Make a tape muzzle about 1 m (3 ft) long for small or medium-sized dogs or 1½ m (4–5ft) for large ones. A well-twisted gauze bandage is the ideal material as it is soft and will not slip. Otherwise you can use a length of sufficiently wide sewing ribbon, or any type of cord or string that is strong, soft and thick enough not to hurt when it is bound tight. Make a simple knot at the mid-point of this tape muzzle and slip it over both jaws tightening it when it is about halfway along the nose (fig. 1).

– Run it under the chin and make another simple knot (fig. 2).

– Take it behind the neck tying two knots to fasten it, and if possible finish it with a bow that can easily be released when needed (fig. 3).

– Make sure the dog does not have its tongue between its teeth when it is applied and that it does not push the tape off with its front feet; keep its head up and feet down.

The illustrations on these pages show the restraining of a dog with a tape muzzle

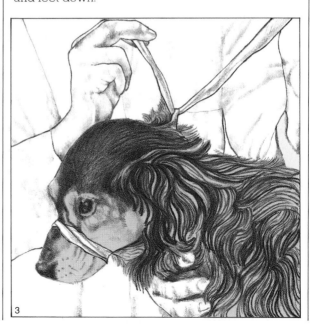

3

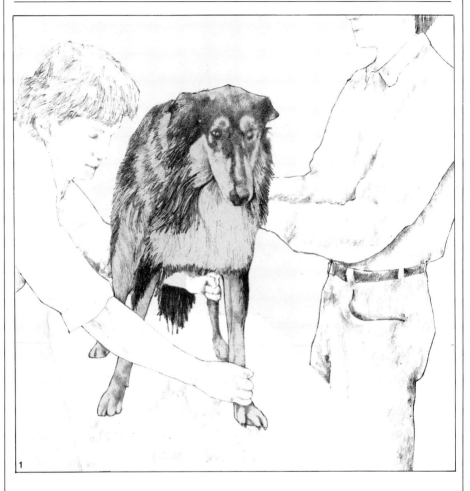

1

1.-2. Restraining a dog:
laying it on its side for access
to abdomen and thorax

A dog should be restrained by a muzzle when:
– you are a stranger to the dog, or, even if you are familiar with it, you cannot foresee its reactions;
– you are about to do something that you know will be painful;
– you are aware that immobilizing the jaws will help to keep the dog still, and allow you to be more confident about handling it, even if the animal is not usually a biter.
A muzzle should not be applied when:
– the dog is tame and patient;
– there are breathing problems;
– the injury is in the mouth or nose area.

■ Restraining the trunk

■ If the size of the dog and the place where it is found permit, it is best placed on to a table of suitable size; you will then be able to stand and adopt a more comfortable and less tiring position in which to restrain it effectively.

If the dog is too big or you are far from home in open country, you will need to keep it still on the ground. Choose a suitable place, preferably in a quiet and sheltered spot, and put the animal on a blanket, sheet or piece of clothing.

First aid is made very much easier if you have the help of another person; the hints given here are directed at the helper who is primarily concerned

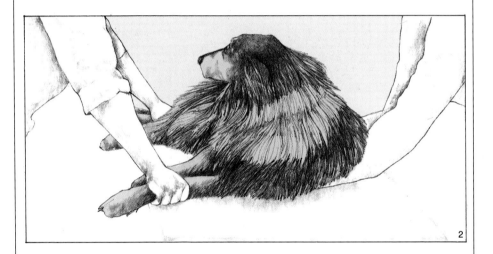

2

with keeping the animal still.

Restraint is achieved in various ways, depending on the part of the body that has to be attended to. The following instructions are best understood in conjunction with the relevant illustration.

Abdomen - Thorax

Lay the dog gently on its uninjured side, getting your helper to support the trunk and moving the legs on that side (fig. 1, 2).

Next, leave the helper to restrain the dog, using one hand to hold the front legs just above the carpus, and pressing the arm on the dog's neck to prevent

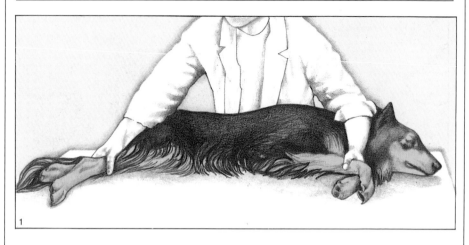

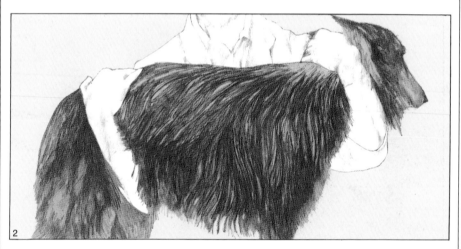

Ways of restraining a dog for access to various parts of the body: 1. abdomen-thorax; 2. back; 3. front leg; 4. front paw

the head from rising; and with the other hand immobilizing the hind legs, holding them above the hock, using that arm to press upon the trunk in front of the hip (fig. 1).

Back

The position shown above in figure 1 would prevent easy access to the back. If you need to treat that area, therefore, the dog must remain standing. It can be prevented from moving by the helper holding it tightly against their own body, with one arm passing under the abdomen just in front of the hind legs and the other round the neck (fig. 2).

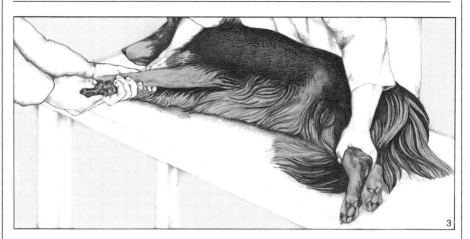

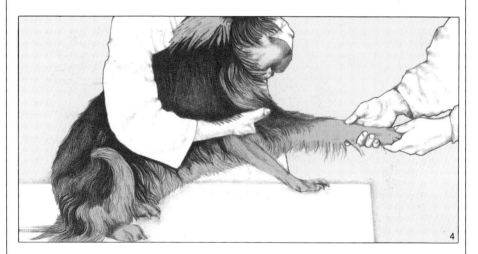

Front leg

Lay the dog down as shown in figures 1 and 2 on pages 26 and 27 and immobilize by holding the hind legs together with one hand and the uninjured front leg with the other, leaving the injured leg free (fig. 3).

Front paw

To treat the front paw the dog, unless very restless, need not be lying down. To prevent the paw from moving, hold the leg behind the elbow with one hand having placed that arm across the animal's back, whilst securing its neck and head with your other hand (fig. 4).

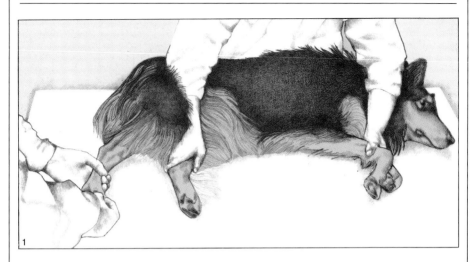

Hind leg

Lay the dog down as in figures 1 and 2, on pages 26 and 27 on the uninjured side leaving the injured leg free; try to keep that leg still by putting the arm that holds the lower (uninjured) hind leg in front of the thigh (fig. 1).

Hind paw

The hind paw is harder to immobilize if the dog is on its feet. Therefore lay the animal down and get a helper to hold the thigh above the knee (stifle joint) with one hand, and the foot above the hock with the other (fig. 2).

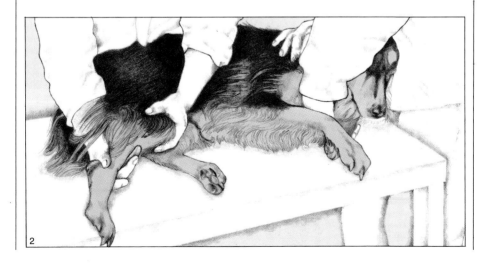

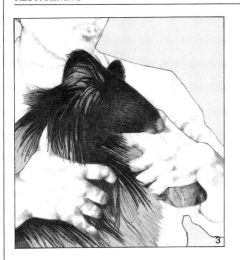

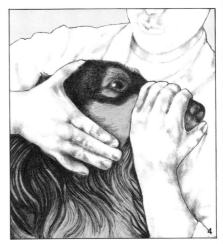

Ear

With the dog standing, hold its nose with one hand grasping it from above and pressing it to yourself, while immobilizing the neck with your other hand, putting your arm tightly around the dog's back and shoulder (fig. 3).

Eye

With the dog standing, use one hand to hold the nose from below and press it to yourself, while your other hand immobilizes the head; holding the skin on the back of the head makes it easier to keep the lids open (fig. 4).

Cats

As the temperament of cats is different from that of dogs, so is the manner of restraining them.

It can be very difficult to give first aid to a cat, especially when it does not want assistance. In fact it is often so good at attack and defense, and so swift and agile that it is impossible to help. As well as immobilizing it, one must get it to co-operate in keeping still. Here are a few suggestions on how to manage this:

Ways of restraining a dog for access to various parts of the body:
1. hind leg
2. hind paw
3. ear
4. eye

– Do not use force unless absolutely necessary: few cats will actually be intimidated, most of them get restless and fight back.

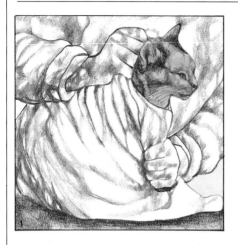 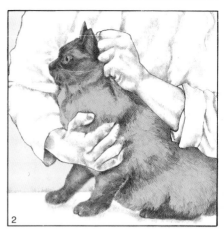

1. Restraining a cat with the aid of a blanket

Restraining a cat for access to various parts of the body:
2. head
3. hind leg
4. front leg
5. trunk

– Wrapping an injured cat in a blanket or towel is a useful procedure if no suitable basket or other container is available and you want to carry it securely. In this way, you will avoid being scratched and the cat will be restrained safely (fig. 1).

– The less excitement involved in immobilizing an injured cat, the better. For this reason, try to involve as few people as possible since they will only upset the cat more.

– Try to keep the cat calm by moving around slowly, without making any undue noise or raising your voice.

– The cat will feel more at ease if you keep the surroundings as quiet as possible by switching off sources of noise, such as television, radio, record players and electric appliances, and also dim the lights.

– Clear a suitable table of any objects, and remove the cloth if there is one, and gently place the cat up on it.

– When immobilizing the cat, avoid restraining it in an unnatural position. It is important to choose a comfortable way of holding it if you want to make it co-operate to any degree.

With one hand grasp it by the scruff (i.e. the loose skin at the back of the neck) firmly taking hold of a good fold of skin as near the head as possible, and with the other hand try to immobilize the body and limbs to allow first aid to be applied to the wound (fig. 2,3,4,5).

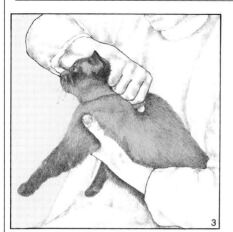

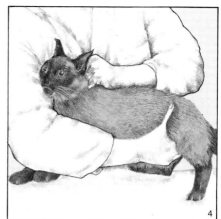

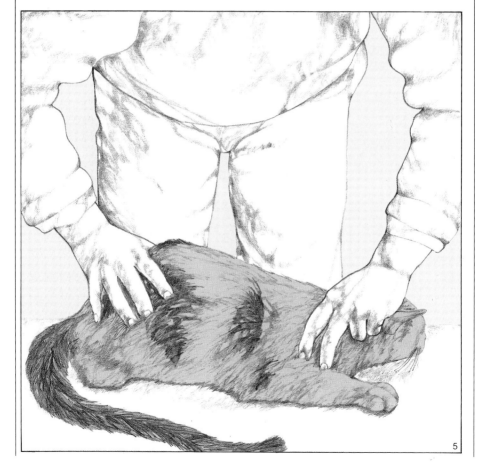

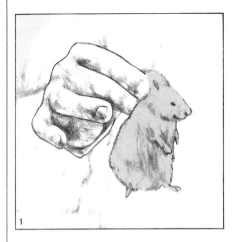

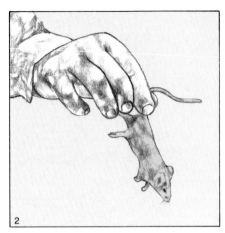

Restraining small mammals
1. by the upper part of
the neck
2. by the end of the tail

Small mammals

■ Leaving aside rabbits and guinea pigs, which are
the larger members of this group and as a general
rule much tamer, small mammals are often hard to
restrain. They can be fairly wild and aggressive,
and may resist even normal handling by moving
suddenly and biting. Many hamsters and squirrels
in their desperate, if unjustified, panic may both suffer and inflict serious injury. Always act carefully
and firmly, avoiding sudden movements and alarming noises.
The animals must be taken from their cages by
holding them firmly by the loose skin of the upper
neck. Take hold of a good fold of the skin with the
hand, or with the fingers if the animal is one of the
smaller species (fig. 1). Picking them up in this way
does not hurt the animal and is safest for the handler
as well. With rabbits and guinea pigs it is important
to support the weight of the body by placing the
free hand underneath the animal.
Next, put the animal on a non-slippery surface so as
to observe it, but maintain your grip. It is best to use
low tables to prevent falls should the animal break
free. Mice and rats may be pinned down by gripping the base of the tail between the fingers (fig. 2)
and resting the animal on the palm of the hand; this
will enable you to keep it calm and quiet.
Squirrels and gerbils must never be seized by the
tail, which is very fragile and may be damaged,

causing serious and painful bleeding. If the animal is too wild, avoid pointless and upsetting fights and take the animal to the vet in its cage.

Birds

■ If you have to pick a bird up to take it out of its cage, try above all to avoid the unnecessary fear and fluttering caused by stretching your hand into the cage. This can be avoided by taking the bird out in the dark. First observe where the bird is, then open the cage door and turn off the light. You can then quietly put your hand inside and capture the bird.

When immobilizing a parrot, it is advisable to protect your hand by means of a glove because with its strong beak it can give you a nasty bite.

The best way of holding a bird in your hand so that it is both safe and secure is shown in figure 3. You should take care not to squeeze too hard as you could easily choke it, nor too gently as equally it could escape.

**3. Restraining small birds:
how to hold them in your hand**

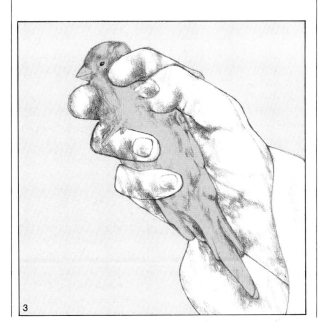

GIVING DRUGS

To work successfully
in collaboration
with a vet, it is vital to
have a good knowledge
of the different ways of
giving drugs and how
to prepare them for use.

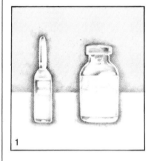 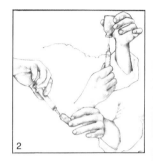

Cats and Dogs

■ **Injections**

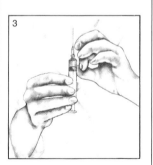

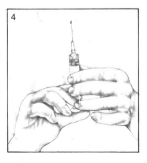

■ Puppies and kittens should ideally be vaccinated to protect them against the common infectious diseases. Your vet will advise you about them and carry out the injections.

Puppies and kittens will generally have a course of injections which will vary in number according to the species and product. These are started within the first 2 to 3 months of life, after immunity acquired from their mother has waned. The animals should be kept away from other cats or dogs, or places where any other cats and dogs have been, until 2 weeks after the last injection of the course has been given. Kittens are routinely vaccinated against feline infectious enteritis (feline panleukopenia) and feline influenza, and puppies against canine distemper, canine viral hepatitis, leptospirosis and parvovirus infection.

These vaccinations will be administered by a veterinary surgeon who after completing the initial course will be able to advise you about the need for further booster injections. Usually, you will only be required to give drugs to animals in the form of pills. However, sometimes, in collaboration with a vet, you might have to give drugs by injection, for example to a dog with diabetes mellitus. We give here a description of the administration of drugs in this way, so that you are aware of this method, too.

Drugs that are given in the form of an injection with a syringe usually come in vials or small bottles with rubber seals (fig. 1).

Often a small serrated file is provided to make it easier to break the glass top; always remember to make at least three cuts around the vial and to use a piece of material or cotton wool to protect your fingers from the glass when you snap the top off. If it is a small bottle, remove the protective cap and clean the rubber seal with antiseptic.

– Insert the needle well into the bottle and draw up the contents (fig. 2). You may notice a certain amount of resistance while emptying bottles with rubber seals. To make it easier to extract the contents, inject a quantity of air before drawing it up into the syringe.

If, while you draw up the medicine, air bubbles form inside the syringe, you should eliminate them as follows:

– point the syringe into the air and pull the plunger back a fraction.
– flick the syringe very lightly with your finger nails until all the air bubbles shift and move to the top (fig. 3).
– push the plunger slowly upwards until the first drop of medicine comes out (fig. 4).

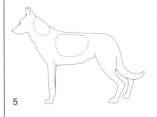

5

Subcutaneous injection:
1.-2.-3.-4. preparation of drug for use
5. recommended injection sites
6. injection into neck area
7. injection into back area

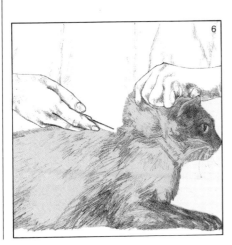

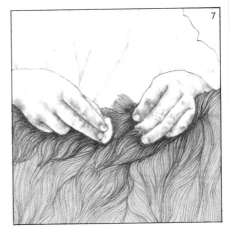

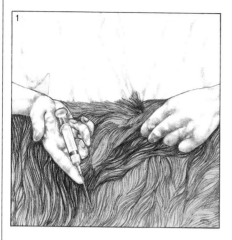

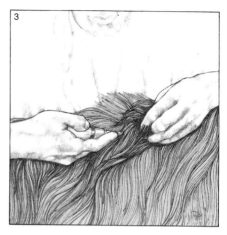

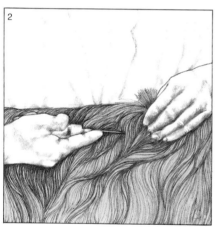

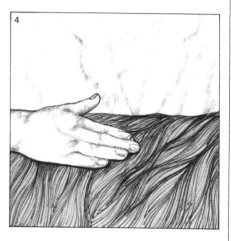

■ Subcutaneous injections

Where to give them

1.-2.-3.-4. Administration of a subcutaneous injection in the back region and subsequent massaging of the site

■ A subcutaneous injection is the easiest way of giving drugs other than by mouth. If they are carried out correctly, such injections need not be painful or dangerous.

Subcutaneous injections are administered into the tissue between the skin and the underlying muscular layer; this tissue is found over all the body but, for practical purposes, the best area is the upper part of the neck and trunk. It is best to avoid injecting over the shoulders and shoulder blades (scapulas) and the central area of the back along the spine as an injection might hit a bone by mistake, especially following a sudden movement on the part of the animal. The areas indicated in the illustration on page 37 (fig. 5) show the safest and most comfortable sites for an injection. The neck region usually has less sensitive and thicker skin, especially in a cat. It is also the ideal site because you can hold the animal still while restraining the head. For this reason, it is the most suitable place to inject into if there is no one else to help (fig. 6, p. 37). In the back region an injection can be easier because the skin is softer but it also allows the dog or cat to move around more freely (fig. 7, p. 37). In this case it is better to have somebody present to assist.

Administration

– Lightly pinch a fold in the chosen area between the thumb and forefinger (fig. 6 and 7, p. 37) and lift it up; make sure there is a definite fold of skin in your hand and disinfect it well with antiseptic, preferably surgical spirit. The spirit, which will soon evaporate, thoroughly cleans the injection site.
– Take the syringe and hold it as shown in the illustration (fig. 1); the forefinger on the needle will make the grip firmer and control the injection through the skin.
– Point the syringe towards the bottom of the fold of skin, slightly angling it and keeping the needle opening facing upwards (fig. 2).
– Push the needle through the skin into the subcutaneous tissue about 1–2 cm (½–¾ in) and then press the plunger down slowly. You may find it difficult to change the position of your fingers so, if your hand is big enough, try to press the plunger in with your palm (fig. 3). The liquid should flow smoothly, unless it is a particularly thick suspension. If it becomes really hard to inject, do not force it. Either pull the needle out a little or push it in a little; if it is still impossible to inject the liquid then remove the needle and begin again.
– After the injection has been completed, massage the injection site thoroughly (fig. 4).

Possible problems

Any subcutaneous injection carried out properly should present no problems.
If the injection goes into the skin and not beneath into the subcutaneous tissue, it can cause local inflammation and a consequential loss of hair which

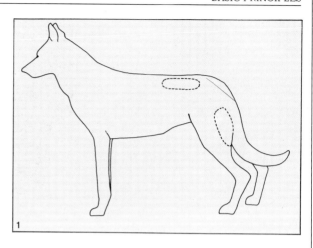

1

will not grow again if the hair follicles are permanently damaged.

■ Intramuscular injections

■ An intramuscular injection has a much faster absorption rate and is used when the drug must take effect in a shorter time.
It is easy to carry out but can present more problems than a subcutaneous injection because the needle is inserted deeper; it is, therefore, particularly important to take care not to harm the nerves or to inject the drug into a blood vessel.

Where to give them

Generally, intramuscular injections are given at the back of the thigh or in the region of the loins in the area shown in figure 1.

– It is best to inject into the muscles of the loins if the drug is irritant to avoid causing any lameness in the leg. However, it can be hard to perform if the animal is thin or of small stature and therefore lacking sufficient muscular tissue.
– Injections into the thigh are those most commonly given, but, because of the risk of damaging the sciatic nerve, you should take great care when choosing the injection site.
You can work out where the best place to inject is by imagining a line joining the knee to the bony edge at the top of the thigh bone (see Anatomical diagram on p. 10); halfway down this line imagine another line that runs perpendicularly to the rear end of the thigh; by

Intramuscular injection:
1.-2. recommended sites
3.-4. how to hold the animal

How to carry out an
intramuscular injection:
5. disinfecting the skin
6. how to hold a syringe

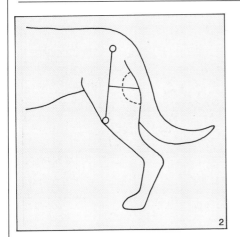

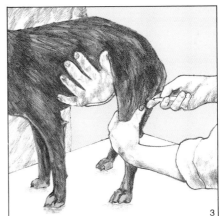

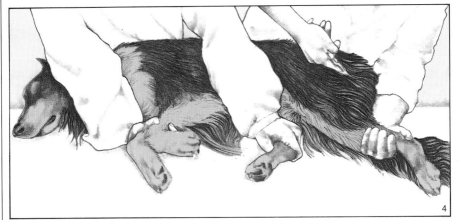

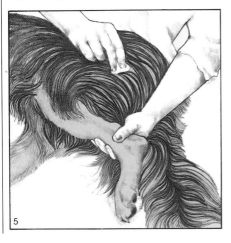

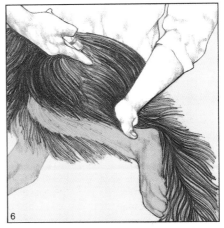

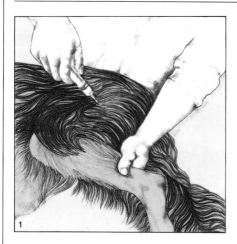
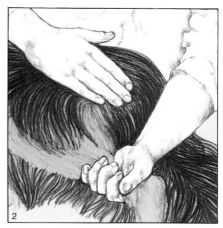

siting the injection along and around the back half of this line, you will not run any risk (fig. 2, p. 41).

Constraining

Intramuscular injections are more difficult to give than subcutaneous ones and you will therefore have to keep a firmer hold on the animal.
Docile cats and dogs are best left standing on all fours with somebody helping to hold their head and body still (fig. 3, p. 41). If, on the other hand, they are too agitated, then they should be laid on their sides and held as shown on pages 26 and 27.
With one hand hold the hind leg in which the injection is to go, placing your hand just above the hock; hold the syringe in the other hand (fig. 4, p. 41).

Administration

– Disinfect the chosen site with a piece of cotton wool dipped in antiseptic, wiping thoroughly (fig. 5, p.41).
– Hold the syringe as illustrated in the drawing (fig. 6, p. 41); if the animal is small and has a slender thigh, control the needle entering the muscle with the forefinger.
– Before inserting the needle, direct the syringe slightly toward the rear end of the thigh. Then, push the needle in about 1–2 cm (½–¾ in), according to the size of the animal. Before pushing on the plunger, withdraw it a little; if nothing comes out into the syringe, the needle is inside a muscle, i.e. it is placed correctly; if you get a little blood flowing into the syringe, then the needle has hit a blood vessel;

How to carry out an
intramuscular injection:
1. inserting the needle
2. massage

the needle must be withdrawn and re-inserted at a different point (fig. 1). Once placed correctly, gently press the plunger in to inject the liquid.
– After the injection, remove the needle and massage the area well (fig. 2).

Possible problems

Damage to the sciatic nerve or to one of its branches, following insertion of the needle at the wrong site or sudden movement by the animal, can cause varying degrees of paralysis of the leg, especially in small-sized cats and dogs.
Injection of the drug into a blood vessel instead of the muscle will bring serious problems if the liquid is a suspension or an oily solution as this can cause blockage of the microscopic blood capillaries. There are also certain drugs that are dangerous if injected directly into the bloodstream.

■ By mouth: tablets, capsules and coated pills

■ Giving tablets and capsules need not be unduly troublesome or painful, but it can be awkward because the animal usually does not co-operate and often tries to resist by refusing to open its mouth and swallow.
To avoid any unnecessary struggle, try to be swift and decisive. It is a good idea to catch the animal by surprise, but do not scare it. Above all, do not let the animal know that you are about to administer its medicine or it may run off and hide. It is surprising how pet animals quickly learn the significance of the preliminary preparations for administering medicines. If a tablet has to be divided into parts, use a sharp knife or razor blade; if the surface is not already scored, cut some grooves on it with the blade before trying to break it to stop it from crumbling. After cutting, remove the traces of surplus of powder on the tablet's edges by tapping it gently and blowing. This will prevent an unpleasant taste lingering in the mouth. In cats, especially, a bitter taste greatly increases salivation and therefore drooling.
While coated tablets are fairly readily swallowed, capsules may stick to the inside of the animal's mouth or to your fingers if they become wet. Uncoated tablets have a rougher surface and may cause problems. A useful tip is to lubricate them with a little "Vaseline" or cooking oil.

Administration

– Take the item to be given between thumb and

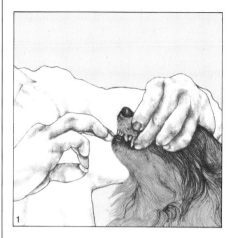

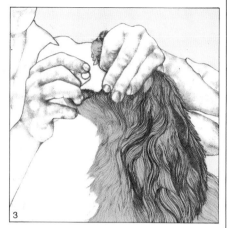

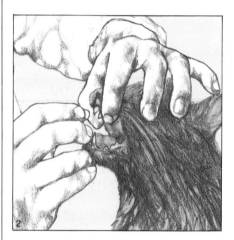

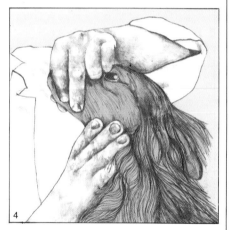

1.-2.-3.-4. The pictures illustrate in sequence how to administer a tablet

index finger of one hand, and with the other hand force the animal to open its mouth as shown: press the upper lips against the teeth using the thumb on one side and the index and middle fingers on the other, just behind the upper canine teeth (fangs). As soon as there is an opening between the incisors, push the jaw down with the middle finger of the hand holding the drug.

– As soon as the mouth is open, push the drug in towards the base of the tongue (fig. 3).

– Close the mouth immediately, lightly supporting the head. To encourage swallowing, lightly tap the chin or stroke the throat from the top downwards;

when you see that the motion of swallowing is beginning, release the head (fig. 4).

If you fail to make the animal swallow the pill, you can:

– either, force the animal to swallow before it can spit the drug out by making it drink some water by means of a syringe or a small glass of water, though it is unlikely you will manage to be quick enough;

– or, give the drug with food, unless this is not recommended and could impair the drug's effect. Capsules and coated pills cannot be divided and may be hidden in a piece of meat, cheese or chocolate after cutting a hole with a knife, or in a ball of minced meat. Tablets can be broken into small bits and mixed with the food, but it is better not to crush them too small to avoid creating an overall unpleasant taste.

5.-6. Administration of liquid medicine using a syringe

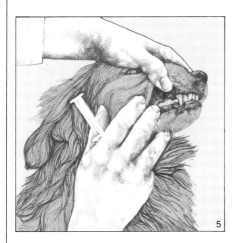
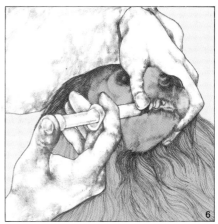

The second solution can be difficult because the animal may have lost its appetite.

■ Syrups and drops by mouth

■ Liquid preparations can be given with a dropper that sometimes comes with them, or with a small bottle or spoon if the animal keeps still and co-operates. However, animals rarely take liquid medicines willingly and have to be persuaded to swallow them.

With cats and most dogs it is easiest to use disposable syringes (without a needle and well washed if previously used) or a dropper to draw up the amount needed.

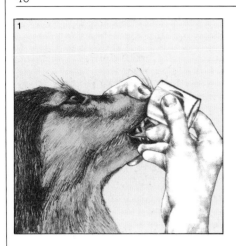

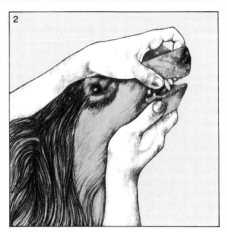

Administration

– Introduce the nozzle of the syringe into the side of the mouth, in the space behind the canine teeth, i.e. between them and the premolars (fig. 5, p. 45). Rest it on the tongue and direct it towards the throat, while lightly supporting the head (fig. 6, p. 45).

– Press the plunger: as soon as the liquid flows, the animal will start to swallow. The administration must be quick but allow the animal to swallow at a normal pace to avoid some of the drug reaching the windpipe and causing coughing. If the animal starts to cough and refuses to co-operate, remove the syringe and repeat the whole procedure more slowly later.

If the dose of liquid is larger, you can try to get the animal to swallow it by using a small beaker or bottle. Trickle it into the side of the mouth sideways inside the cheek, using the lower lip as a funnel (fig. 1). This will only work with dogs, and then only with tolerant ones. If the dog refuses to swallow and stores the fluid in the cheek as in a bag, raise its head and slightly open its teeth to cause a flow toward the throat (fig. 2).

■ **Applying medication to the eyes**

■ Before applying medication to the eyes, make sure the eyes are clean. If, inside or around the edge of the eyelids, there are sticky discharges like mucus or pus, or crusts from their drying, wash the eyes gently and carefully.

■ **Cleaning the eyes**

■ To clean the eyes:
– It is best to use a wad of clean gauze, preferably

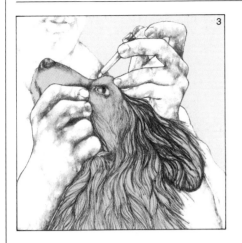

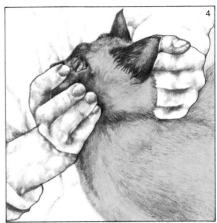

1.-2. Giving medicine with a
small beaker
3. Application of eye drops
4. Application of eye ointment

sterilized; cotton wool, though soft, can lose fibers
and is therefore less suitable.
Moisten the gauze with an eye wash (boric acid
lotion or similar, available from pharmacists in small
bottles). It is preferable not to use tap water but if
this is inevitable, use tepid, not hot or cold.
– Pass the moistened gauze gently over the eyes
a few times, moving from the side nearest the nose
outwards.
– Wipe the lids with dry gauze, a clean cloth or
some kitchen roll; never use dry cotton wool.

■ **Applying eye drops**

■ Raise the animal's head with one hand, holding
the nose between thumb and index finger while
exposing the inside of the lower lid with the middle
finger. With the other hand, hold the dropper or
squeezy bottle and let it release one or two drops into
the eye; a larger amount tends to trickle out of the eye
and would be wasted. You should keep a distance of
about 2 cm (¾ in) between the tip of the dropper or
bottle and the eye, to avoid sudden movements
resulting in injury to the surface of the eye (fig. 3).

■ **Applying eye
ointment**

■ Apply a ribbon of ointment about 3–5 cm (1–2 in)
long on the inner edge of the lower lid; the animal
will blink and so spread it uniformly over the eye
surface. Putting the tube directly into the eye can
be risky as the animal might very well move; if
this is the case, it is simpler and safer to apply it
using the tip of the index finger (well washed), as in

figure 4 (p. 47). With the middle finger of the same hand, turn down the edge of the lid for easier application.

■ **Ear preparations**

■ Ear preparations usually take the form of drops to be put into the ear canal or creams and lotions to be applied to the ear flap.
Before treating the ear you should always make sure the ear is clean. The presence of wax, which may have dried to a crust, can act as a barrier rendering the drug ineffective. You can check to see if wax is present by examining the ear canal, with the help of a torch if needs be (fig. 1).

■ **Cleaning the ear and applying the medication**

■ The ear canal must be cleaned gently, especially if the lining is inflamed. There is little risk of hurting the ear drum, given the shape of the outer ear of a dog and cat (see Anatomical diagram on p. 16), especially if you have somebody to help hold the animal still properly (see p. 31) and you apply the medication correctly.
There are many products available for cleaning the ears of animals. You can use one recommended by the vet or use some drops of the actual preparation prescribed as medication to clean the ear first and then add some more. Liquid paraffin is also very effective for this purpose.

To clean the ear:
– With one hand hold up the ear flap so you can see the opening of the canal, and with the other allow some drops to fall in. Avoid letting the tip of the bottle or dropper touch the canal lining (fig. 2).
– Massage near the base of the ear a few times to help to spread the liquid inside (fig. 3).
– Wait a few minutes to allow wax or crusts to soften.
– First clean the vertical part of the canal (see Anatomical diagram on p. 16) using a good quality cotton bud which will not lose the bud during use (fig. 4).
Move from the bottom up along the walls of the canal, keeping the cotton bud vertical and pushing it in as far as the shape of the ear allows: when the bud reaches the bend that separates the horizontal part of the canal from the vertical part, it will go no further.
In cleaning the outer part of the canal and the flap

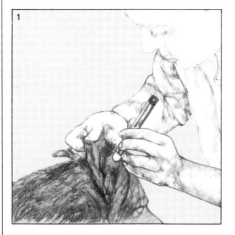

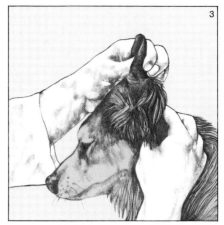

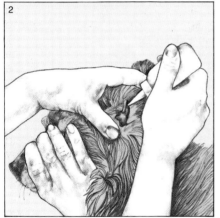

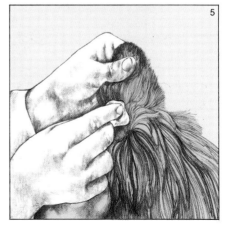

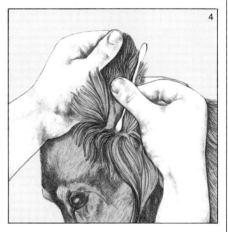

Cleaning the ear:
1. examination with the aid of
a small torch; 2. administering
preparations; 3. massage;
4. cleaning with cotton bud;
5. cleaning with a piece of
cotton wool

you can simply use a piece of cotton gauze or cotton wool wound round a finger (fig. 5, p. 49).

After cleaning, introduce the ear drops according to the amount and frequency prescribed. Two to five drops are usually needed, depending on the preparation and the animal's size.

■ Mouthwashes

■ Dogs and cats cannot easily be made to use a mouthwash or gargle with solutions in an effective way. If really necessary, it is easier, therefore, to apply solutions directly to the gums. However, there are only a few indications for their use.

Administration

– Use gauze in wads of several layers or well folded a few times; wind this around the index finger to form a covering and keep it in place with the thumb (fig. 1).

– Dip the index finger into the mouthwash until the wad is saturated (fig. 2).

– Run the index finger gently over the gums, slowly

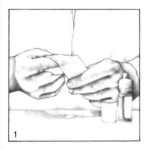

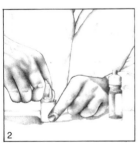

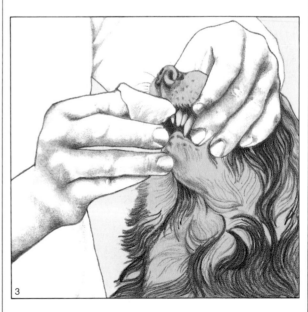

massaging them from the tooth margin outwards and from front to back (fig. 3).

■ Cleaning the teeth

■ In both dogs and cats, bacterial plaque forms at the junction between the gums and the teeth (it looks like a yellowish-grey crust). In this plaque mineral salts are deposited that come from the saliva, forming a crust that is hard and foul smelling, called tartar.

Gradually this layer of tartar spreads and thickens, inflaming the gums and causing them slowly to recede (see fig. 1 and 2 on p. 224). The speed at which tartar will form varies between animals, depending on individual factors, diet and species. In any case, it is advisable to clean the teeth at least once a week. If this is correctly done, teeth will remain strong and healthy. It will lessen the risk of abscesses involving the roots, inflamed gums, and the bad breath which seems to develop with age.

As cleaning teeth is such a fastidious job, animals do not like it, especially restless and impatient ones, and particularly cats. The best way is to just clean the teeth calmly and firmly and gradually get the animal used to it. Start when the animal is

1.-2.-3. Applying a mouthwash to the gums with gauze 4.-5. Preparing a toothbrush for cleaning an animal's teeth

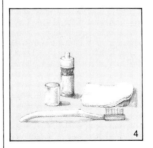
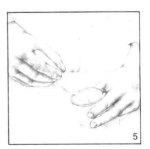

about 6-7 months old, when the final teeth are in place.

Teeth can be cleaned in one of two ways:
1. Take a child's toothbrush with soft nylon bristles (fig. 4) and moisten it in an antiseptic mouthwash, perhaps recommended by the vet, or just in tepid water containing sodium bicarbonate (1 teaspoonful in half a glass of water) (fig. 5).
Move gently over the teeth with a rotary motion, pressing on the part nearest the gum and on the teeth most readily covered in tartar (canines and

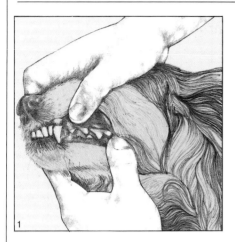

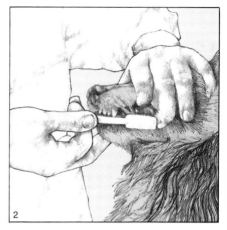

upper incisors, premolars and molars) (fig. 1 and 2).
2. If the animal will not co-operate or if it is simply
too difficult because the animal's mouth is too small
or unsuited, you can clean the teeth quite effectively with gauze prepared as described on page
50. Premolars and molars are more easily reached
with the finger and massage will be better tolerated
as it is gentler than a brush (fig. 3).

Whichever method you choose, take care not to get
your finger bitten.

Cleaning the teeth:
1.-2. with toothbrush
3. with gauze

Opposite:
administering preparations
to small rodents:
4. by mouth
5. by subcutaneous injection

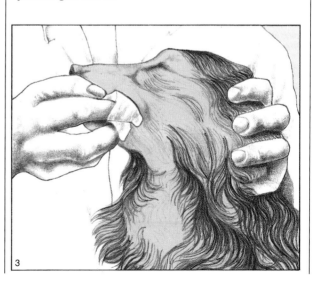

Small mammals

■ Giving medicines by mouth

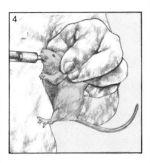

■ Giving liquids by mouth is relatively easy with the larger species such as rabbits and guinea pigs: follow the same procedure as with small cats, introducing the preparation into the mouth with the aid of a teaspoon or, best of all, a syringe without the needle. With the smaller species, which are difficult to catch and hold still, the task becomes more of a problem. Squirrels, hamsters and gerbils will fight and it will take two people to give the medicine. One should restrain the animal, as explained on page 34, and the other should administer the preparation with a very small (1 ml) syringe (fig. 4).

■ Applying ointments and lotions

■ Use of ointments and lotions should be restricted to cases of extreme need because rodents clean themselves continually with their tongues and are likely to swallow some of the preparation.

■ Injections

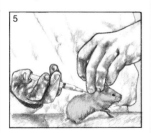

■ Subcutaneous injections on rabbits or guinea pigs are easy to perform and present no problems. It is much harder to inject the smallest mammals subcutaneously; the most suitable place for these, however, would again be the fold of skin on the neck. Bear in mind that the skin is surprisingly resistant to the needle entering (fig. 5).

Birds

■ Giving medicine by mouth

■ This is the most common and suitable way of administering medicines to birds. The preparation should be mixed with water, food or food pellets according to the manufacturer's instructions. If the bird is very ill and cannot eat or drink, the preparation must be given with a dropper or syringe (without an attached needle) inserted inside the beak, which is then held as closed as possible.

■ Inhalants

■ This method involves the bird inhaling a medicine in the form of a vapour in cases of lung infection or parasitism (respiratory acariasis). Place the bird in a small cage totally enclosed within a plastic bag in which the inhalant can vaporize for 15–20 minutes.

TAKING THE BODY TEMPERATURE

The normal temperature of cats and dogs is 38.5°C (101.5°F). It may be a bit higher or lower depending on individual variation. You should take the rectal temperature as it is the easiest to measure and the only significant one. Choose a moment when the animal is quiet (not following exercise or when the animal is excited) and, to have an accurate reading, take the temperature three times in a day.

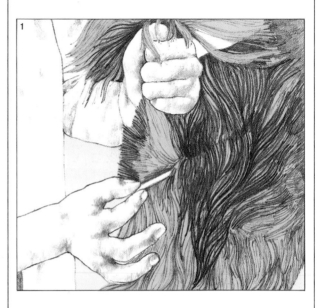

■ **Thermometer**

■ It is best to use a prismatic thermometer and it must be a clinical one. In some the bulb is long, in others short and squat: the former are easier to insert; the latter tend to be stronger and therefore more resistant.

■ **Measurement**

■ If insertion is difficult, especially with cats, lubricate the instrument with "Vaseline," cooking oil or liquid paraffin. Insert it gently to a depth of 2 cm (¾ in) or slightly more if it is a large dog. Then you must wait a couple of minutes before removing it (fig. 1).

■ **Assessment**

■ A temperature reading between 38.5°C (101.5°F) and 39°C (102–102.5°F) is not significant. Beyond 39°C (102.5–103°F), there is a high temperature, 40–42°C (105°F upwards) a serious fever. Below 38°C (100°F) we have hypothermia, a general cooling of the body; this happens in some pathological conditions such as severe shock, exposure, and in bitches prior to whelping. In puppies and kittens body temperature is normally a fraction (0.5°F) higher than in adults.

1. Taking the rectal temperature

FIRST-AID BOX

A small and well-stocked first-aid box should be at hand in every pet owner's home, and during trips and outings by car, to allow prompt help using the correct materials in any emergency. Fully stocked boxes for human use can be bought, but it is a good idea to know what should be present and prepare a box yourself.

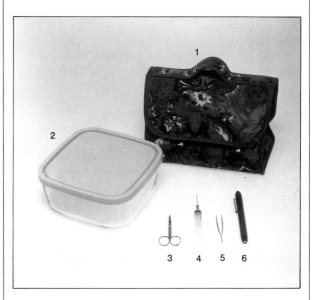

■ **Case**

■ **Instruments**

Material in illustration:
1. Sponge bag
2. Plastic freezer box
3. Scissors, curved on flat with rounded points
4. Syringe
5. Tweezers
6. Electric torch

■ The container must be light, strong, easy to carry and preferably watertight; a large sponge bag or a plastic freezer box with airtight lid are both cheap and effective solutions.

■ The instruments must be good-quality ones. Clean and disinfect them periodically to ensure that there is no rust or dirt.

Tweezers
For extracting thorns, foreign bodies in ear, nose and eye, or fragments of soil and other contaminating material in wounds. The best type is a pair with narrow but rounded points. They are easily obtainable from pharmacists.

Scissors
These are indispensable for cutting gauze and plasters, and removing hair around wounds; those curved on flat and with rounded points are safer and easier to handle. They can be found at pharmacists.

Syringes
For giving drops where needed, and for spraying deep wounds with antiseptic. Keep two pre-sterilized disposable 5ml ones ready for use.

Small torch
For examining ears, mouths or wounds. Must be slimline and easy to hold, with well-focused beam. From electrical suppliers.

■ Material to stop bleeding

■ There are a few items you can have ready in case of severe bleeding.

Tourniquets
To reduce severe haemorrhage in limbs. They can be bought from pharmacists, but ordinary wide elastic will do if at least 30 cm (1 ft) long and sturdy enough. Tourniquets should only be used in cases of extreme need and then for the shortest time possible (maximum 15 minutes).

Ice pack
Handy and not bulky, ensuring a cooling source even in summer for about 10 minutes. Useful for stopping bleeding and also for bruises and sprains or heatstroke. Available from pharmacists.

■ Antiseptics

■ These must have good cleansing power and, above all, they should not sting to avoid the animal reacting. They are available as liquids and can thus be poured into smaller containers that are lighter and less bulky. Suitable ones are bottles with droppers that have contained eye or ear drops, once washed out thoroughly.

Hydrogen peroxide
Good for disinfecting abrasions and surface wounds, especially when infected with earth, rust or plant fragments, since it reduces the danger of tetanus spores.

Organic iodine solutions
These will not sting and they disinfect efficiently. Dilute in water to wash deep or dirty wounds, and apply neat after cleaning.

■ Material for treatment

1. Cotton wool
2. Re-freezable ice pack
3. Antiseptics
4. Adhesive plasters
5. Bottle with dropper
6. Tourniquet
7. Gauze pads
8. Gauze bandages

Bandages. Two or three gauze bandages 5–7.5 cm (2–3 in) wide.

Gauze. Packs of sterile gauze containing one or several layers.

Sticking plaster. A reel of sticking plaster (preferably fabric-based) 3–5 cm (1–2 in) wide. This can be cut into strips of the length desired.

Cotton wool. Packed in a roll rather than loose in balls.

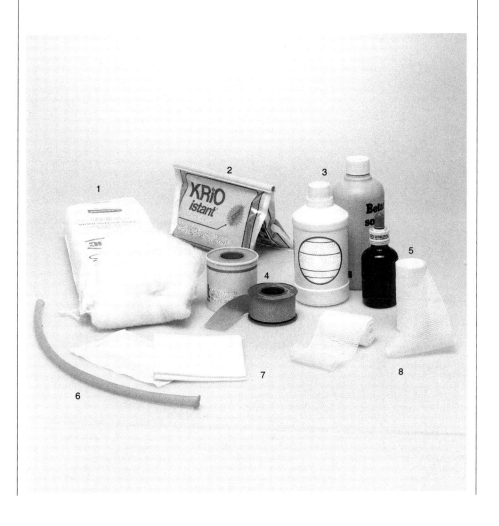

FIRST AID
FOR
CATS AND DOGS

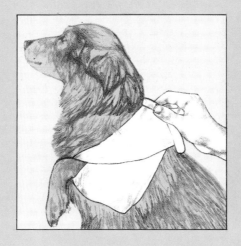

INJURIES

SKIN INJURIES

FRACTURES, DISLOCATIONS, SPRAINS

SERIOUS INJURIES

EYE INJURIES

EAR INJURIES

NOSE INJURIES

SKIN INJURIES

The cases that most often call for first-aid intervention are skin injuries. In this chapter we deal with injuries to the body's surface, other than ears, eyes and nose, which will be dealt with in separate chapters.

CAUSES

★ **Cuts.** These are the most frequent causes of injuries to the skin.
Fragments of glass, wood splinters, nails and other sharp metallic objects scattered on the ground or at the bottom of ponds, river beds, lakes or on shores often injure the paws.
Similarly, thorny bushes, wire fences and barbed wire, are potentially dangerous, damaging especially the trunk and neck.
More rarely we find cuts being caused by various domestic and garden tools, such as knives, axes or hedge clippers.

★ **Bites.** These result from fights between dogs or cats, the latter especially in the breeding season; they mostly occur on the neck, shoulders and flanks.

★ **Shots.** As a result of hunting accidents, the shooting of trespassing animals or malicious damage.

★ **External wounds following serious injuries.** When animals are hit by cars, or fall from great heights, these will often accompany fractures and internal lesions.

ASSESSMENT

To assess how grave an injury is, you must carefully examine the size and depth to discover the severity of the wound.

• **Extent**

• It is easier to assess the extent of the injury if it is in a hairless area or on an animal with a short coat. Otherwise, with a long coat, the hair must be parted and, if necessary, cut away and foreign bodies removed to reveal the size of the injury (as illustrated in fig. 1).

• **Depth**

• The depth of the wound usually shows how serious it is, in that not only the skin but deeper parts may be involved as well, such as underlying blood vessels, nerves, tendons, muscles and even organs in the thoracic and abdominal cavity.

Assessment of extent of
wound in long-coated animals

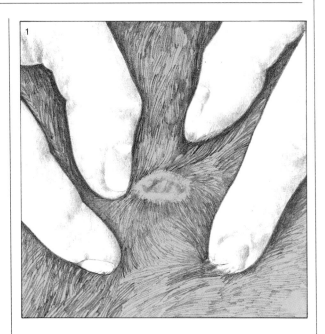

Abrasions

These are the most superficial form of skin injury, since they affect only surface layers without penetrating the skin to any great depth (fig. 1a on the next page). However, they are usually the most extensive and the most painful. In most cases very little blood flows, as only the capillaries within the skin are harmed.

Surface wounds

In the case of a surface wound the skin is cut, but the structures below are undamaged, and blood flow (fig. 1b on the next page) is slight and soon stops, since only small vessels at the center of the skin are cut.
What sets an abrasion apart from a skin wound of any depth is the edges: in abrasions the cuts have no clear edges and are more scrape lesions; in skin wounds the sides of the cut can clearly be moved apart.

Deep wounds

Where wounds are deeper, there may well be subcutaneous damage of a more serious nature (fig. 1c on the next page).

Cut vein

This produces strong, steady bleeding of dark red

Schematic diagram of skin
with lesions of varying depth
(see Anatomical diagram on
p. 19):
a. Abrasion
b. Surface wound
c. Deep wound

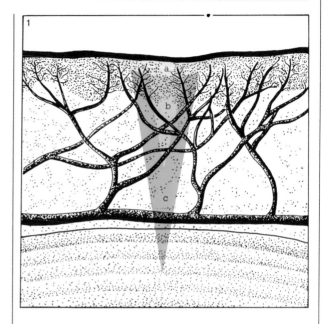

blood. The seriousness depends on the size of the vessel; if the vein is of small or medium size, bleeding may stop automatically.

Cut artery

A cut artery is less common than a cut vein. It will produce swift and heavy bleeding of bright red blood. It is generally harder to stop the haemorrhage, though this will depend on the size of the vessel involved.

Injuries to nerves and tendons

Injuries to nerves and tendons are harder to assess but may potentially result in paralysis or difficulty in moving the affected joints.

• Sites

• The sites of injuries that can prove most dangerous are:

Neck

Lesions of the windpipe on the underside of the neck can impede breathing and admit air under the skin which swells and crackles when palpated. If the jugular vein or carotid artery (lying alongside the windpipe) is cut, bleeding becomes very serious. It is unlikely that any first-aid measure will effect a remedy.

Potentially dangerous areas
for skin injuries:
a. Neck
b. Thorax
c. Abdomen
d. Foreleg
e. Hind leg

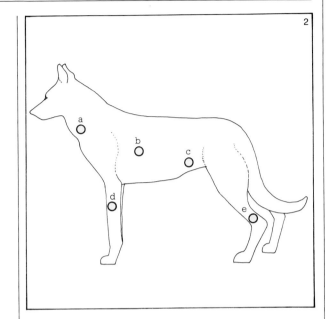

Thorax

If a cat or dog suffers a wound at a point where the rib cage is not protected by the shoulder or back muscles, the lung could be penetrated and damaged. This can result in severe injuries, usually allowing air to enter the pleural cavity (pneumothorax) and cause the lung(s) to collapse.

Abdomen

Deep wounds in the abdominal area, above all along the underside where the muscles of the wall are thin, can penetrate the abdominal cavity and damage the organs within.
If the opening of the wound is wide, the abdominal organs may spill out.

Foreleg

Between the elbow and the paw on the front of the leg there are large superficial veins. These will bleed heavily when they are cut.

Hind leg

On the hind leg possible injury sites are above the hock at the back, where the Achilles tendon may be damaged, and just above the hock on the side where there is a vulnerable vein very near the surface.

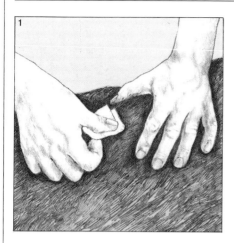 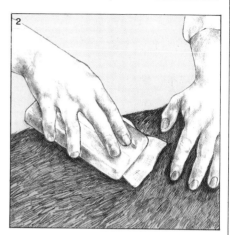

TREATMENT

■ **Checking bleeding**

Checking bleeding:
1. by manual pressure
2. by cooling

■ In the case of superficial wounds, or deep ones not involving sizeable vessels, the blood loss should be slight. The bleeding can therefore usually be stopped by simply applying constant pressure for some minutes (fig. 1).
Use a pad of sterile gauze, a folded handkerchief or a clean cloth. If at all possible, avoid fabrics, such as wool, which may irritate and leave fibers.
If after two minutes blood still oozes, cool the wound with an ice pack. Put a gauze or clean cloth between the wound and the cooling source while keeping up steady pressure until bleeding stops (fig. 2).

If you see that the bleeding is swift, copious and unstoppable, you should apply a tourniquet to check it until the vet arrives. Make use of the tourniquet following the advice on page 68.

Material illustrated opposite:
1. Rubber strip cut from an inner tube
2. Gauze bandage
3. Twisted strip of cloth
4. Laces
5. Nylon stockings
6. Tourniquet
7. Strong elastic bands
8. Braces

Proper tourniquets can be bought in pharmacists, often with velcro fastenings to ensure correct tightness. If no rubber tourniquet is available, other soft and elastic materials that will not hurt the skin will serve (large elastic bands, strips of inner tube, short braces, elastic belts etc.).
As a last resort any strong fastening could be used (string of a suitable size, shoe laces, strips of fabric).

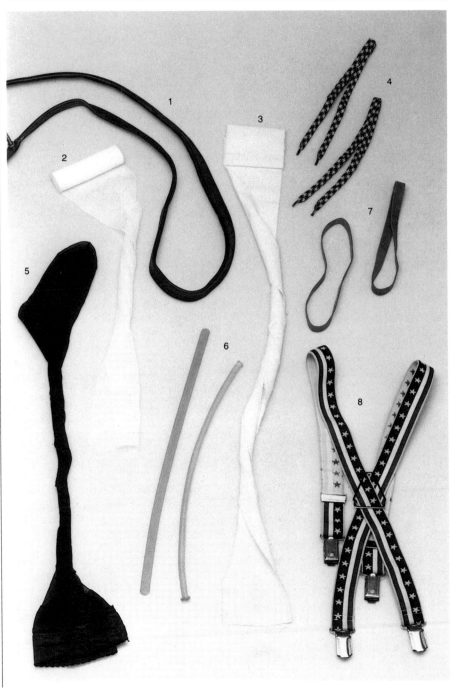

1. The figure shows the points at which tourniquets may be applied

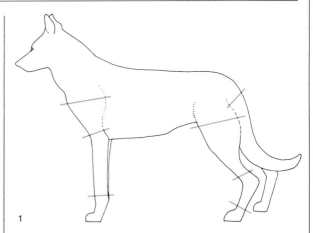

1

■ Applying a tourniquet

■ Tourniquets can only be used for lesions to limbs or tail. They should be applied only at the points shown in figure 1 on the legs and tail, never around the neck.
– Wind the tourniquet round the spot chosen and tie a simple knot.
– Then, tighten it until bleeding slows down sufficiently.

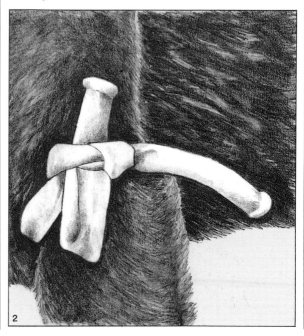

2. Example of knot for tying a tourniquet.

2

– Rather than tying a double knot, form a firm bow for easy untying (fig. 2).

– In order to tighten and slacken the tourniquet efficiently, you can then insert a stick under the strap and twist as necessary.

Do not leave the tourniquet in place for more than 15 minutes, then slacken off to restore circulation to tissues. If necessary, you can re-apply it.

Bleeding cannot always be stopped completely; in such cases, continue to apply pressure and cooling even after applying the tourniquet.

■ Cutting the fur

■ Before cleaning and disinfecting the wound, cut away surrounding fur with scissors (curved nail scissors if possible) as in figure 3.

Begin at the edges of the wound, taking care the hairs do not fall into it (use gauze or a piece of clean cloth to protect the wound). Clear 1 cm (½ in) around the edges, thinning the surrounding coat if this is long.

■ Cleaning and disinfecting

■ For this, it is best to use non-alcoholic fluids, to avoid excessive stinging which will further upset the animal.

3. Removing the hairs around the wound

Antiseptics

Use mild antiseptic lotions to clean and disinfect but avoid stinging with strong solutions. Products such as antiseptic creams are suitable as they clean and disinfect. For superficial wounds soiled with earth or produced by plants (thorns, pointed branches) or rusty metal, apply hydrogen peroxide to reduce the risk of tetanus spores infecting the wound.

Cleaning

If a superficial wound is dirty with mud, dust, saliva after bites, or other matter, it must be cleaned up to prevent any infection.
Superficial wounds should be cleaned with sterile gauze or a cloth moistened with antiseptic diluted in lukewarm water (fig. 1). Do not use absorbent cotton wool which may leave fibers in the wound (fig. 1).

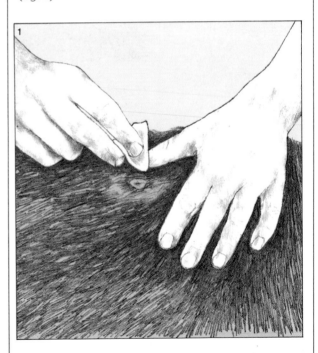

1. Cleaning a superficial wound

For deep wounds, it is a good idea to use large syringes of 5, 10 or 20 ml if you have them, to spray water or diluted antiseptic into the cavity of the wound and flush out any debris (fig. 2).
If the injured part is on the extremity of a limb, place it into a bowl or basin.

2. Cleaning deep wounds

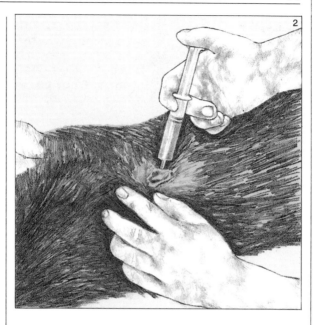

Drying

Make sure the wound is clean and then dry the coat with a clean cloth, towel or kitchen roll.

Disinfection

Apply the same antiseptic, diluted according to the manufacturer's instructions, pouring a fair bit into the wound and round the edges, and spreading it by lightly dabbing with gauze (fig. 3).

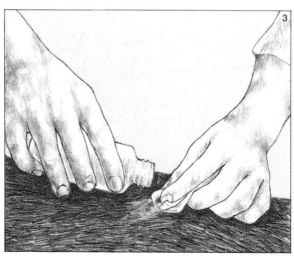

3. Disinfection of the wound

Protecting the wound

To keep the wound clean, or prevent further damage or bleeding through movement of the part, it is best to protect it with a bandage.
There are different ways of applying a bandage to the different parts of the body in order to ensure that it is effective and will not slip.

Appropriate material for protecting the wound

– Pads of gauze, preferably pre-sterilized; or small pieces of cloth like handkerchiefs, provided they are clean. These are put directly on the wound for immediate protection.

– Gauze bandages 5–10 cm (2–4 in) wide, depending on the part. These can be replaced by strips of cloth from sheets, towels or cotton garments. A bandage around the wound will keep the gauze pad in place, give added protection and keep the edges of the wound together.

Material illustrated opposite:
1. Scarf made of light fabric
2. Handkerchiefs
3. Shirt sleeve
4. Gauze pads
5. Gauze bandages
6. Sticking tape
7. Sticking plaster
8. Strips of cloth
9. Tea cloth

– Sticking plaster 1–3 cm (½–1¼ in) wide, to fix the bandage; if there is no surgical plaster, use normal household sticking tape, or split the end of the bandage lengthwise for about 20 cm (8 in) or more, forming two strips to be wound round and tied together.

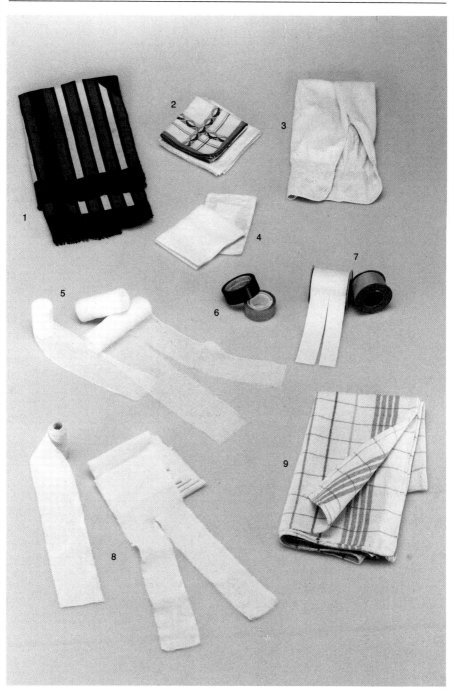

Injuries to the feet

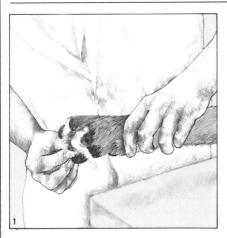

1. Put cotton wool wads between the digits, but do not touch the wounds with dry cotton wool

2. Apply a gauze pad to the wound

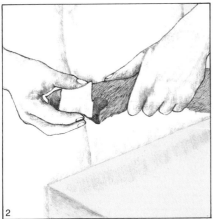

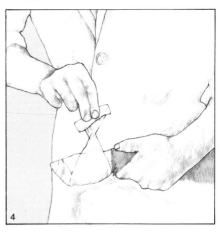

3. Wind the bandage around the paw beyond the carpal or tarsal pad (the largest pad in the center of the paw)

4. To make the bandage more secure, twist it every two or three turns

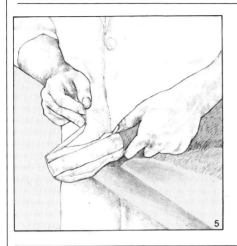

5. Apply a strip of adhesive tape along the sides of the bandaged area running from top to bottom

6. A further strip of plaster is placed around the upper edge of the bandage, overlapping so as to make it partly stick to the haircoat

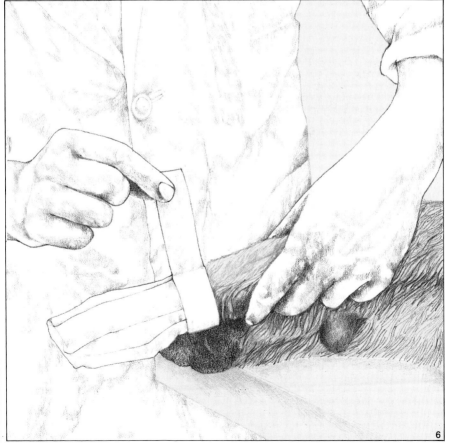

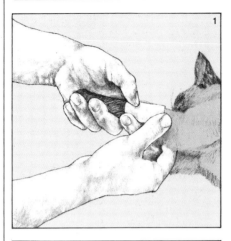

Foreleg and hind leg

1. Apply a pad of gauze to the wound

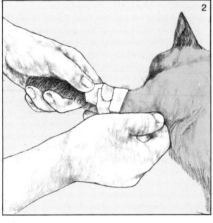

2. Fix the gauze with a strip of adhesive plaster to prevent it slipping

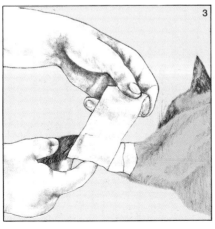

3. Wind the bandage around the paw until there are at least three layers of gauze

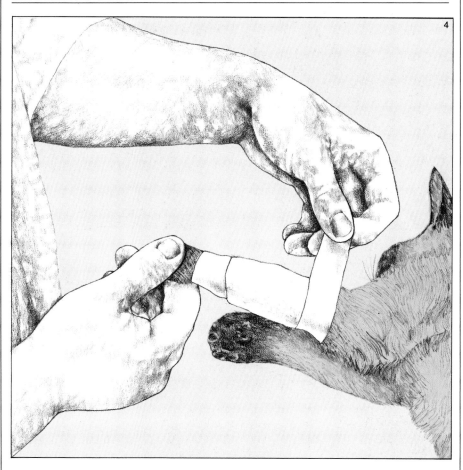

4. Fix the bandage at both ends with a strip of adhesive plaster making it stick partly to the haircoat

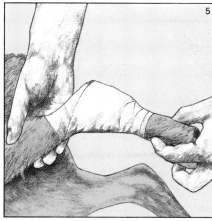

5. For wounds near a joint, include the joint itself within the bandaged area

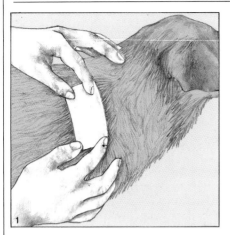

Neck and shoulder

1. Put a gauze pad over the wound and fix it with a strip of adhesive plaster if necessary

2. Wind the bandage several times around the neck and thorax

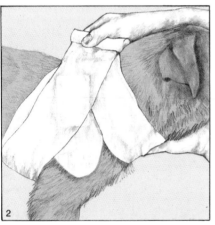

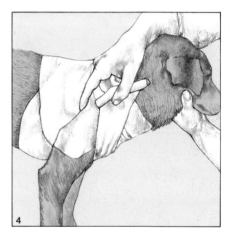

3. Take the bandage across the back and between the front legs

4. Secure the bandaging after at least three or four runs across the injured spot

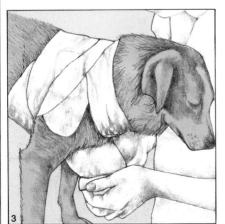

5. Fix the front edge of the bandage by winding round adhesive plaster, partly sticking it to the haircoat

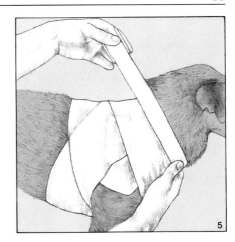

6. Fix the back edge similarly

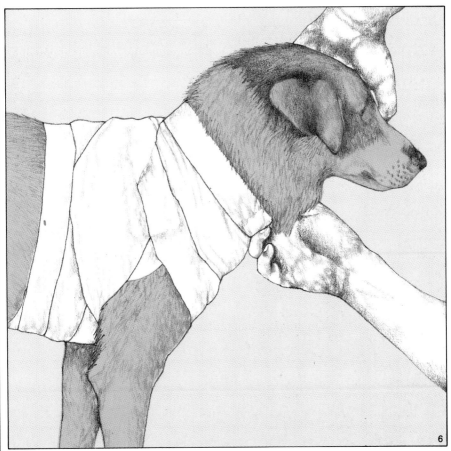

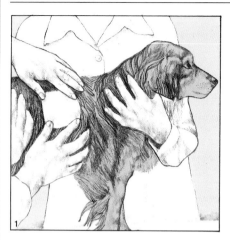

Thorax and abdomen

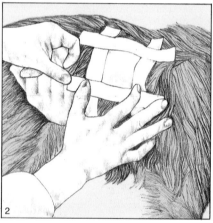

1. Apply a gauze pad over the wound

2. Fix the pad with strips of adhesive plaster to attach it to the haircoat

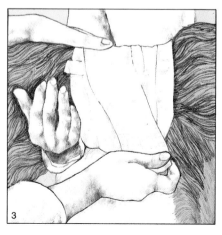

3. Wind the bandage over the pad for several turns

4. Fix the end of the bandage with a piece of adhesive plaster and wind two more strips around each edge of the bandage so that it sticks partly to the haircoat

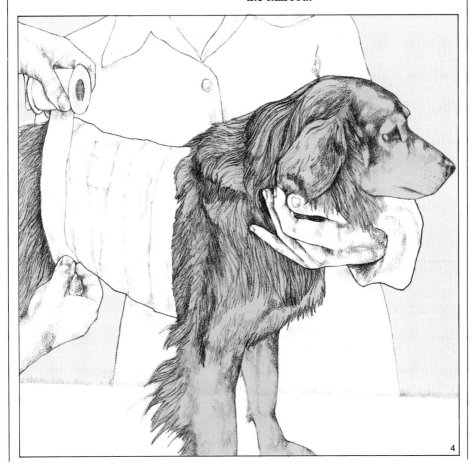

4

Thighs

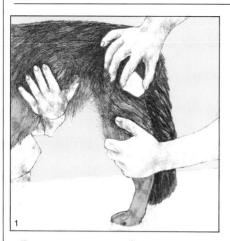

1. Apply a gauze pad to the wound

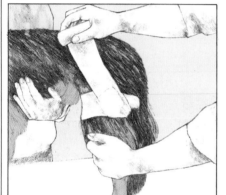

2. Fix the pad by winding a bandage around the injured area

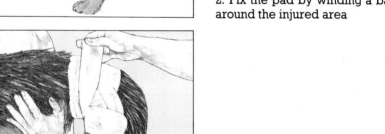

3. To prevent the bandage from slipping, include thigh, flanks and abdomen

4. Fix the bandage with two adhesive plaster strips applied to its edges and make them stick partly to the haircoat

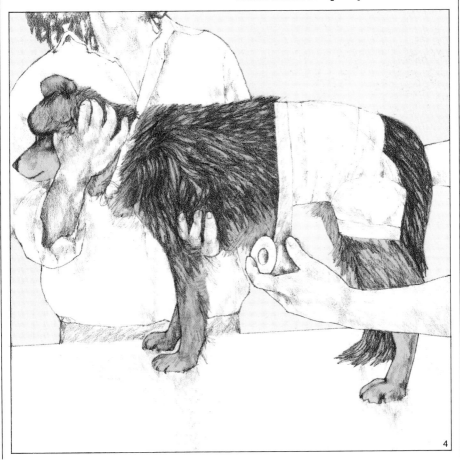

4

FRACTURES, DISLOCATIONS, SPRAINS

Fractures, dislocations and sprains are the result of injuries to bones and joints.

CAUSES

★ **Collision with motor vehicles.** This is the most common cause.
★ **Falls from windows, balconies, flat roofs.** Frequent accidents with cats and puppies.
★ **Running into objects or awkward movements.** During play, running or in scuffles.
★ **Kicks and other blows.**

ASSESSMENT

● **Fractures**

● A fracture means that the bone is broken. The many ways in which this may occur can be roughly categorized as follows:

Complete fracture

The bone is severed into at least two parts (fig. 1)

Multiple fracture

The bone is broken in several places and into pieces of different size. In general this produces severe injuries. It is the worst kind of bone fracture to repair (fig. 2).

Partial fracture

The bone is cracked but not completely broken, remaining in one piece (fig. 3). In puppies and kittens, whose bones are more elastic because they are not yet fully calcified, fractures can be of a special type called "greenstick" fractures, so-called because they resemble a young twig splitting when it is bent (fig. 4).

● **Dislocations**

● Here the ends of the two bones which form a joint are separated, following severe damage to the ligaments that normally hold them together (fig. 5).

● **Sprains**

● Sprains constitute rather less serious injuries in which the ligaments of a joint are stretched or torn, though without being completely severed so that the joint remains intact.

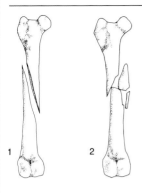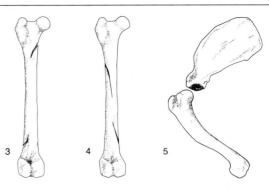

1. Complete fracture
2. Multiple fracture
3. Partial fracture
4. "Greenstick" fracture
5. Dislocations

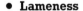

● **Lameness**

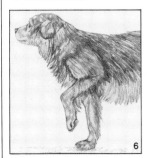

6. Behaviour indicating pain
in a joint: lameness

To distinguish between the lesions described is often difficult for a pet owner. For a precise assessment of the severity and type of lesion, you should therefore have the animal examined by a veterinary surgeon as soon as possible.

Nevertheless, one should have some idea of how to recognize a bone or joint injury and to estimate how serious it is.

This helps in deciding what, if any, measures to take so as to limit the consequences that often follow such damage.

First of all, it is important to note whether one or more of the signs described here are present.

● The cause of lameness is the pain that moving or carrying weight produces at the point of injury. It may be hardly noticeable and merely consist of a restricted and hesitant movement of the limb, or the limb may be virtually unused and held up most of the time instead of being placed on the ground. You will find that the animal will not remain in its normal standing position (fig. 6).

Lameness in itself does not tell us what is wrong, but reveals the presence of damage that is causing pain.

If the lameness is slight, you should wait and see if, some hours after the accident, matters improve; if so, there may have been severe pain initially which disappears soon afterwards, showing that the damage was very slight.

If, however, you find the animal continues to be lame, even slightly, then you should consult a vet about the problem.

• Swelling of the limb and deformity

• To assess whether the limb is at all swollen, compare it with the opposite, normal one. A marked deformation of a joint could indicate a dislocation (fig. 1).

• Twisting of the limb

• If there has been a fracture somewhere along a bone, the limb is often twisted upwards, downwards or to the side, showing that the leg has been completely broken. If you are not sure, compare the shape of the injured limb with the opposite, normal one (fig. 2).

• Shortened limb

• Complete fracture of the thigh bone (femur) or the humerus causing an overlap of the two ends, or a severe dislocation of their upper joints (hip or shoulder) can make the limb appear short, and thick at the top. Sometimes it looks as if it is hanging and, as the animal moves, it swings freely (fig. 3).

• Exposed fractures

• We speak of a fracture as being exposed if the end of the broken bone pushes through muscles and skin and is visible. This is a serious outcome and requires instant attention from a vet to prevent the exposed part from becoming infected (fig. 4).

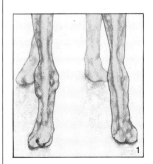

If there is lameness without obvious signs of injury, try to find its site by palpating the limb systematically and carefully. If, at a certain point, this causes repeated pain, it is best to restrict movement of the animal by following the advice in the chapter on restraining (p.24).

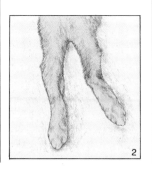

– First handle and inspect the spaces between the digital pads and the tarsal or carpal pad, since lameness often comes from wounds, foreign bodies or severe skin irritation in these areas (fig. 5).

– Next, examine the joints starting from the digits (toes) and moving upwards. Try to see whether they are swollen and painful, squeezing them lightly between thumb and index finger (fig. 6). Then try to make them flex and extend, observing whether they move easily and whether the movement causes any distress or pain, or produces a grating sound.

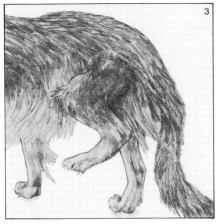

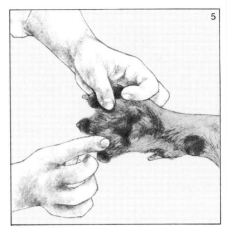

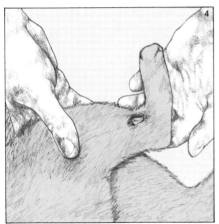

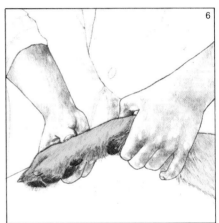

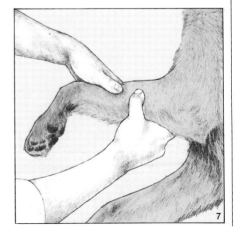

1. Deformed joint
2. Twisting of the leg
3. Shortened limb
4. Exposed fracture
5. Palpating and examining digits
6. Palpating the joints
7. Ascertaining that bones are in one piece

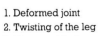

– Make sure the bones are in one piece (fig. 7 on previous page) by palpating them all the way along from one joint to the next, trying to note swellings or bone deformities, signs of pain or any noise caused by the ends of fractured bones rubbing together.

TREATMENT

If you suspect that the cat or dog has suffered a bone or joint injury, it would be advisable to have the animal seen by a vet at once.

■ **Immobilization of limb**

■ In the case of a clearly serious injury, it may help to immobilize the limb at once with a splint; for example, if you are dealing with a complete fracture or obvious dislocation, or if you are in a remote spot and the animal, being too big to carry, has to walk.

Appropriate material

– Gauze bandages for binding up the injured area. These could be replaced by strips of cloth from garments, towels or sheets, or handkerchiefs if the limb is small.
– Cotton wool for making a pad to prevent the splint from directly touching the injured and painful part. Failing this, one may use pieces of soft material, in a single layer if thick enough, or folded several times (e.g. the sleeve of a woollen pullover, a piece of blanket or similar); if you are out in the countryside, a bundle of grass stems or hay will do, so long as it is soft.
– Splints. The size required varies according to the part to be immobilized, from 15–20 cm (6–8 in) to 40 cm (18 in) and more. They must be flat and rectangular in cross section, strong and yet light. The best material is wood, especially if light and resistant; you can also use lolly sticks, slats from fruit boxes or straight bits of branches split lengthwise.
If nothing else is at hand, you can use plastic objects such as tubing of an appropriate diameter (e.g. electrical conduit or water pipes) and cut into halves; newspaper or corrugated cardboard to wind round the limb are also a good substitute.
– Adhesive plasters, shoe laces, string, bandages, to fix the splints.

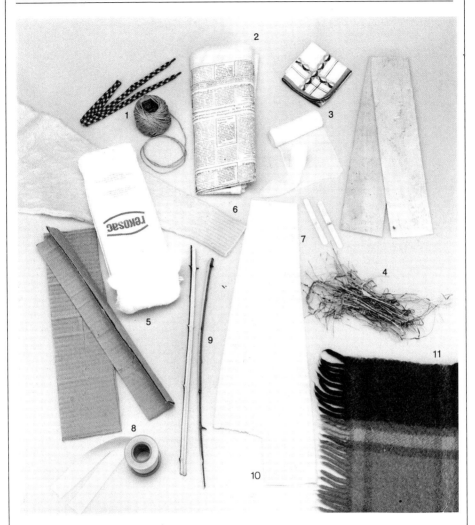

1. String and laces
2. Newspaper
3. Handkerchief and gauze
4. Sticks and straw
5. Cotton wool
6. Pullover sleeve
7. Lolly sticks
8. Cardboard and plaster
9. Branch split lengthwise
10. Strip of cloth
11. Strip of blanket

Immobilization and splints

The ways of immobilizing limbs vary according to the part injured.

While ideally the aid of a vet should be sought, in cases of extreme emergency an example of immobilization outlined here could be followed. These methods are not the only possibilities; they are aimed at giving a guideline to the principles of immobilization.

The foot and the forearm

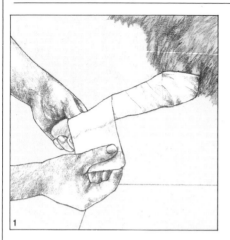

1. Bandage the limb with a gauze bandage or long strips of cloth

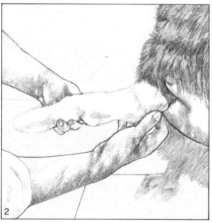

2. Wind a layer of cotton wool around the bandage. To make it stay in place better, a further bandage may be laid on top of the cotton wool

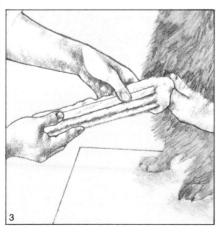

3. Apply 3 splints of suitable length round the limb, one each side and one below

4. Fix the splints with two or more strips of adhesive plaster or tape

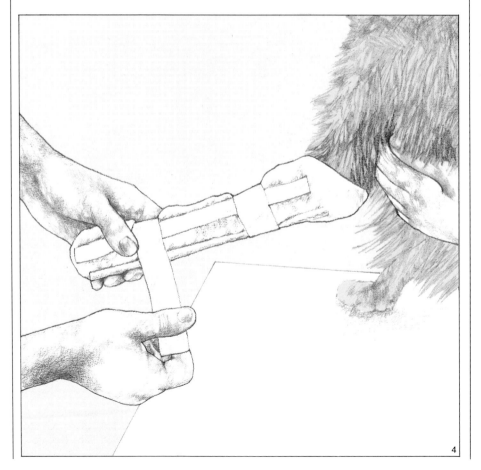

4

Hind leg: leg and hock

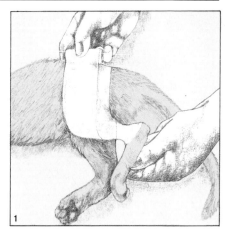

1. Bandage the limb with a gauze bandage or long strips of cloth. To prevent slipping, pass them round the flanks and abdomen as well

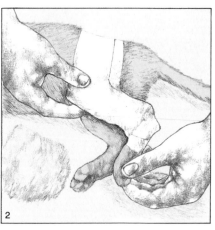

2. Wind a layer of cotton wool around the bandage. To make it secure, add another bandage on top

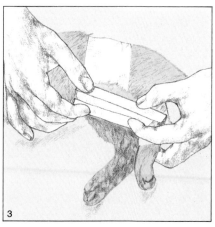

3. Apply 3 splints of suitable length to the limb, one in front, and one on each side

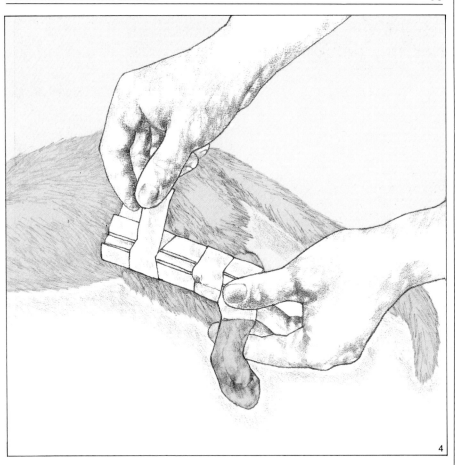

4

4. Fix the splints with two or more lengths of adhesive plaster or tape

Forelimb: elbow, arm and shoulder

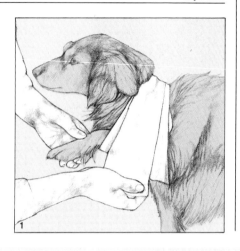

Hind limb: Knee and thigh bone

1. In cats and small dogs we can use a crutch of thick wire, moulded as shown in the figure and joined with adhesive plaster or tape. The part to be supported must be padded with soft material such as cotton wool fixed with gauze bandages.

Apply the crutch by extending the limb and fixing it with strips of plaster. For better adhesion wind strips of adhesive tape round the crutch at the points where it is to be fixed to the limb with other tape

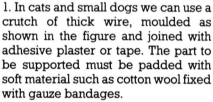

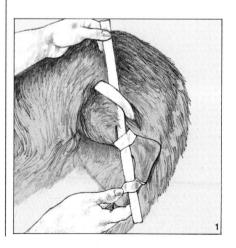

2. For medium-sized or large dogs use a splint fixed to the limb by adhesive plaster at the points shown in the figure, inserting pieces of cotton wool between splint and limb.

This effectively immobilizes the knee and hock. To restrict movement of the thigh will require additional bandaging over the splint as explained on page 82

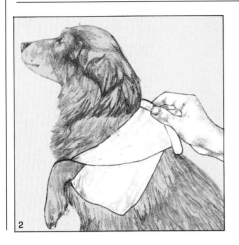

1. Wind two gauze bandages or long strips of suitably wide cloth around the neck and injured limb, from top to bottom. The limb should be flexed and held against the chest

2. To prevent the animal from extending the limb, reverse the direction of bandaging after a few turns, passing the bandage in front of the paw. The bandage should then be fixed in the usual way with plaster or adhesive tape

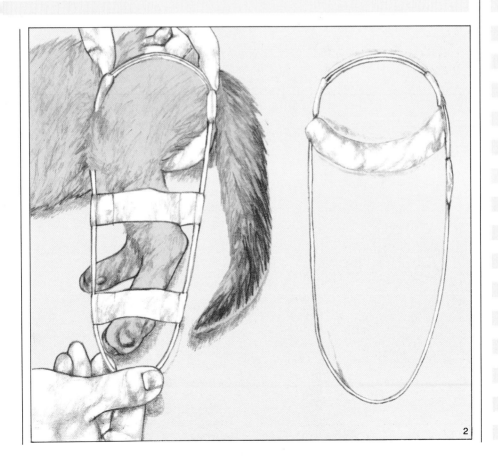

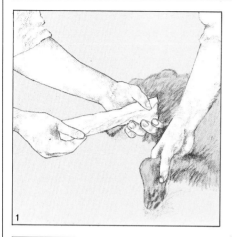

Improvised splints

■ Even if you have no bandages, strips of adhesive tape or cotton wool, you can still immobilize a limb in an effective way for the time being, by using material you will readily find around you in the countryside.

1. Wind a handkerchief or piece of cloth around the limb

2. Gather a bundle of grass or hay suitably long and soft and arrange it around the limb

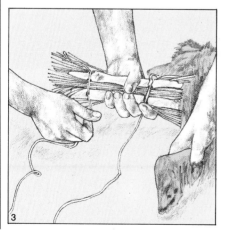

3. As splints, use three sticks split lengthwise and apply the flat side to the pad. With a knife cut two sets of grooves to hold the string with which the splints will be fixed

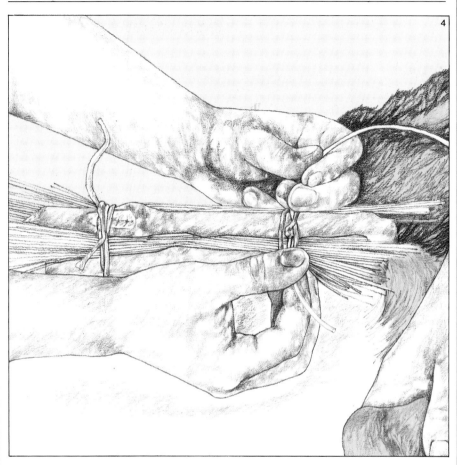

4. Wind two pieces of string or strips of cloth around the splints and tie them after two or three turns

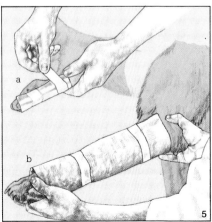

5. Alternatively, use things like corrugated cardboard folded lengthwise (a) or newspaper wound round the limb (b)

SERIOUS INJURIES

W hen an animal is
so badly hurt
that it suffers not only
wounds and bone
injuries, but also serious
damage to blood
vessels and internal
organs, it may be close
to death. In such cases,
you must concern
yourself with giving
vital initial first aid but,
above all, ensuring
swift transportation to a
veterinary surgeon.

CAUSES

★ **Collision with motor vehicles.** How serious the
damage is hinges on many factors (size of animal,
type and speed of vehicle, and the part of it that hit
the animal).
This is the most common cause of death from injury
in animals and it is important to try and prevent it.
Train your dog to obey commands and keep it on a
lead. Do not allow it to wander alone. As to cats, you
can only protect them from dangerous traffic by
keeping them in.

★ **Falls from great heights.** These generally
involve cats or puppies falling from windows, down
stairwells, off roofs or out of trees. How grave the
damage is hinges on the animal's weight, height of
fall (at over 8–10m [25–30 ft] i.e. 2–3 stories, serious
damage is very likely).

★ **Other common causes.** Fights between animals, forceful blows, firearm accidents or mishaps
with dangerous tools (chain saws, motor mowers
etc.). Always be on the lookout for other possible
causes (escalators, glass doors, open washing
machines, accidents with fireworks etc.) and take
measures to prevent serious accidents.

ASSESSMENT

● **To check if the
animal is still alive**

● When an animal is badly hurt, the first thing to
ascertain is whether it is still alive. This is easy if
there is spontaneous movement but can be hard if
the animal is completely still. In this case look for the
following signs.

Breathing movements

In animals, you can examine for signs of breathing
by seeing if there are slight rises and falls of the
chest, abdomen and the last ribs; often these can be
very slow and slight, and therefore difficult to see
with any certainty.

Heartbeat

The heartbeat is felt by putting your hand or
finger tips, depending on the size of the animal,

1. Checking heart beat

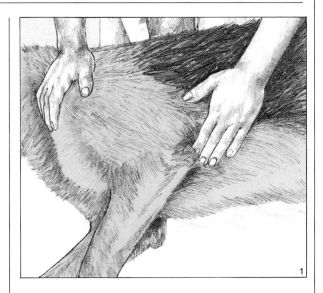

on the left side of the chest behind the elbow joint as shown in figure 1. In this area you will be able to feel beneath the ribs a rhythmic pulse corresponding to the heartbeat.

Arterial pulse

In animals this is felt in the femoral artery by placing the index, middle finger and ring finger together on the inside of the thigh (fig. 2).

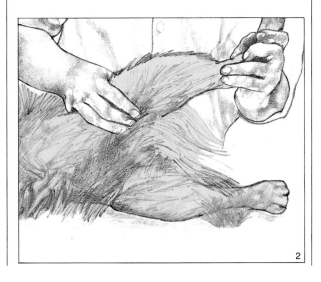

2. Detecting the arterial pulse

In the central part of the inner thigh there is a depression between the muscles running vertically, near the upper part of which you will feel the beat with your finger tips.

● **Assessment of the state of consciousness**

● If the animal is alive it may be lying still in shock. You should then establish whether it is conscious or not.

Response to call

Call the animal and see if it moves its head or eyes, even if only slightly; dogs sometimes wag their tail a little.

Assessment of vision

Pass a hand in front of the animal's eyes about 20 cm (8 in) away and try to see whether they follow your movement. If not, make a quick movement of the hand towards each eye, stopping just short of the lids, without touching the eyelashes. If the animal has conscious vision it will react by closing the eyelids (response to threat, fig. 1).

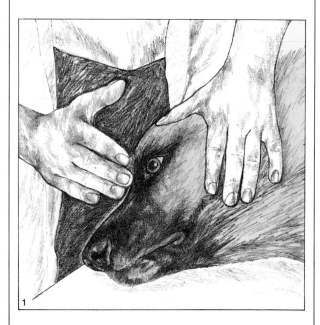

● **Serious state of coma**

● If you have found the animal is unconscious, you should assess how serious this is, namely whether the animal is suffering from the grave depression of brain activity called "coma." This can be done by observing the reflexes of the eyes and the state of the pupils.

Corneal reflex

Lightly touch the corneal surface with your finger (fig. 2).
The normal reaction would be the eye shutting at once. The absence of this reflex in an animal, even if the stimulus is repeated, indicates that it is in a serious state of brain depression.

Light reflex

Take an electric torch and point it at the animal's eye with the beam well-focused on the pupil.
In normal conditions the stimulation of strong light will cause the pupil to contract. If you can see this does not occur, there is probably serious brain depression.
This test is similar to the previous one, but is harder to assess, especially if the surroundings are well lit (fig. 3).

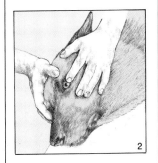

1. Response to threat
2. Observing corneal reflex
3. Observing the light reflex

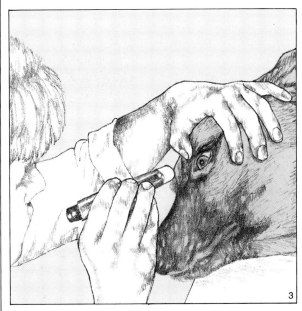

Diameter of pupils

This is easier to observe and varies with the intensity of light reaching the eye: strong light produces a strong contraction of the pupils, whereas darkness

1. Diagram of size of pupil in cats (right) and dogs (left)
a) mydriasis (dilation of pupil)
b) normal pupil size
c) myosis (contraction of pupil)

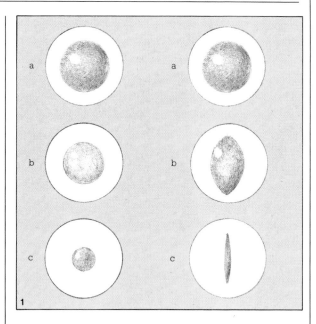

will cause dilation. In daylight without strong illumination (such as sunlight, or strong artificial light) the pupil is of medium diameter.

Carefully examine the eye and if you find contraction (myosis) or dilation (mydriasis) of the pupil in an animal after a serious injury, particularly if it is present in one eye only, this can indicate brain injury (fig. 1).

• External examination

• Having established whether the animal is alive and conscious, you should assess the extent of its injuries by a rapid external examination for wounds or fractures.

While you examine the animal, try to avoid unnecessary movements and carry out unavoidable ones very gently.

Do not forget to inspect the abdomen for possible wounds in the abdominal wall; if the injury is very serious and the viscera have protruded, it will be clearly evident.

• Assessing mobility of limbs

• Before starting to move the animal, it helps to carry out a series of checks to determine whether it is able to move its limbs.

2. Observing the bending
reflex
3. Palpating the spinal column

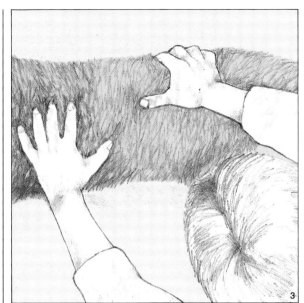

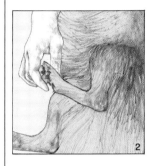

Voluntary movements

If the animal is conscious, observe the limbs and try to discern voluntary movements.

Pedal reflex

If you cannot be sure, then movement can be provoked by the pedal reflex. This is easy to test: simply squeeze the largest (carpal or tarsal) pad or a digit of the paw, or pinch the skin between the digits with some force; if the stimulus is strong enough, the animal normally withdraws its paw (fig. 2). Try this on all four limbs. If you find the hind limbs or the forelimbs are immobile or insensitive, the spinal column may well be damaged.

● Examination and spinal palpation

● Serious damage to the vertebrae can sometimes be detected by simply observing the back and carrying out a gentle examination of the spine. Gently palpate the sharp vertebral projections, which you will feel as small bony bumps along the center of the spine (fig. 3). If you observe hollows, steps or lateral deviations, it might mean a fracture or a bad dislocation of the spinal column. However, much will depend on the animal's position and condition so, if you suspect something unusual, seek an expert opinion immediately.

TREATMENT

■ After an accident, above all, remember that a badly hurt animal will be in shock and that this lowers blood pressure.
Try to think of the comfort of the animal. If the accident happens in cold weather, bring the animal into a warm place with good air circulation as soon as possible.
Similarly if the outside temperature is high, find a cool and ventilated place.
If the animal is unconscious or finds breathing difficult, lay it down on its side extending its head and opening its mouth for easier breathing.
Check that the tongue is not too far back and, if it is, pull it gently forwards out of the mouth (fig. 1).

1. Correct position of head and tongue in a badly injured animal

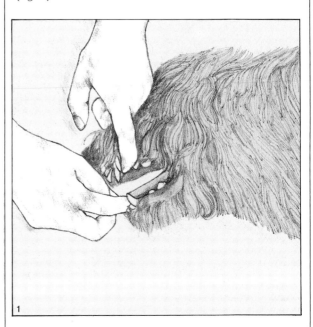

■ Carry out only essential first aid and treat wounds or fractures (see first-aid measures on pp. 62 and 84) only as described in the following cases.
– If the wounds are large and dirty, clean and disinfect them, unless the injury is so serious that there is no time or possibility of doing this.

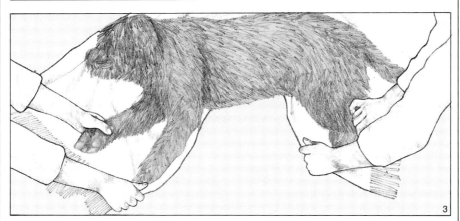

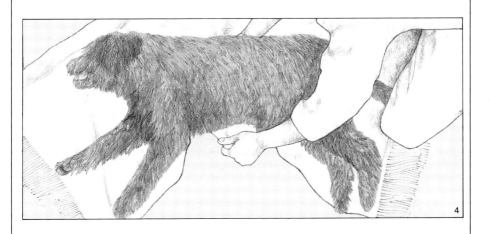

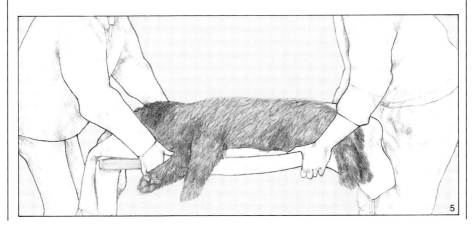

EYE INJURIES

he eyes are a very vulnerable part in animals. The results of an injury are often made worse by a lack of prompt first aid.

Eyelid injuries

As the eyelids are the best protection for the eyes against external attack, they are consequently often injured.

CAUSES

★ **Bites or scratches.** As a result of fights with other animals.
★ **Cuts.** From thorny bushes or sharp objects.
★ **Blows.**

ASSESSMENT

● Carefully check the upper and lower lids for injury or bleeding. Also examine the visible parts of the eye and the third eyelid. This is exposed by very gently pressing on the eyeball through the covering of the upper lid (fig. 1), though this is a task

1. How the third eyelid in cats and dogs is exposed. It is situated at the corner of the eye nearest the nose

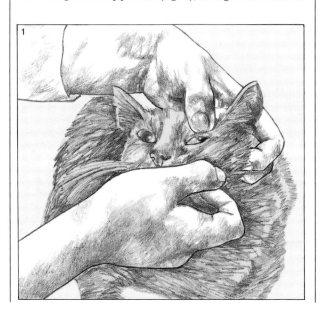

best left to the vet if you do not feel confident.

● **Bruising**

● Because the lids are highly vascular, they are quite often bruised, producing slight bleeding under the skin.

● **Grazes**

● Sometimes the skin of the lid may be merely grazed. This will cause slight hair loss and bleeding.

● **Deep wounds**

● Injuries to the eyelid can also be much deeper and be visible as tears in the skin. You should assess not only the depth but also the extent and, in particular, the site of any damage. Tears to the margin of the lid are more serious both as regards the animal's appearance and the interference with the function of the lids.

TREATMENT

■ If you find there is slight bleeding under the skin or a bleeding wound, put cold compresses over the eye for a few minutes. Use a pad of gauze or cloth folded several times and dip it into clean water as required (fig. 2).
An ice pack may be used, but apply it to the eye only at intervals, to prevent excessive cooling. Take care not to apply ice directly on to the surface of the eyeball as this will stick and cause irreparable damage.

■ Abrasions are cleaned with gauze and antiseptic. Take care not to let any antiseptic go into the animal's eye. Use a non-alcoholic antiseptic which will not sting and hurt the animal.

■ Lesions of the eyelid, especially if deep and extensive or involving the margin, must receive prompt attention from the vet, who may decide to stitch them.
If there will be some delay before a vet can help, clean the wound with boracic acid solution or another antiseptic solution for the eyes, and protect the eye in the meantime by bandaging it as illustrated on pages 110-111.

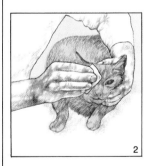

2

2. Applying cold compresses to the eye

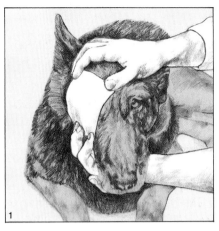

Bandaging the eye

1. Apply a pad of gauze to the eye

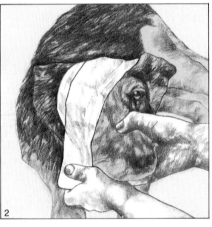

2. Use a gauze bandage or a crêpe bandage to cover the pad and pass in turn around the neck and behind the opposite ear

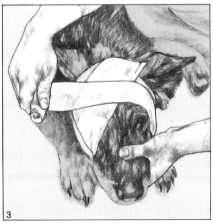

3. After a few turns of bandage in the direction shown, pass the bandage between the healthy eye and the ear on the opposite side. Cross over the bandage and make two more turns around the head

4. Secure the bandage with a piece of adhesive plaster

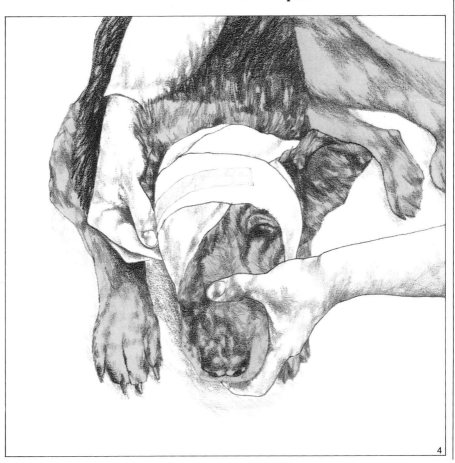

4

Corneal wounds and abrasions

The cornea is the part of the eye most prone to injury, being protected in front only by the eyelids. Corneal injury is most common in cats and dogs with large protruding eyes (e.g. Pekingese).

CAUSES

* **Accidental cuts.** Caused by glass, sharp bits of metal, wood splinters, thorns etc.
* **Cat scratches.** Scratches are the common result of fights with cats.
* **Other common causes.** Injury from blows and car accidents.

ASSESSMENT

● The mildest form of injury to the cornea is an abrasion (fig. 1a), which involves only the outer part. Wounds that cut deeper into the eye look like lacerations (fig. 1b); if it is completely pierced (fig. 1c),

1. Corneal wounds:
a) abrasion
b) laceration
c) pierced cornea

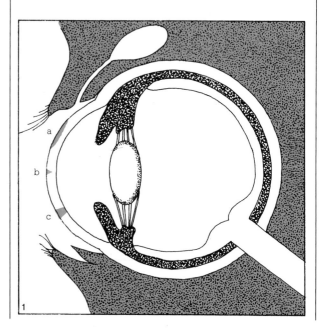

the liquid in front of the lens may escape (see Anatomical diagram on p. 15) and even part of the iris may protrude if the cut is wide enough.

● **Corneal abrasions**

● Corneal abrasion is hard to detect because the cornea is transparent.
You should suspect there might be a corneal abrasion if the animal is greatly troubled by the injured eye. You will notice constant blinking and watering of the eye. Often the eye will become very red.
A vet will be able to assess the situation by applying special stains.

● **Corneal wounds**

● Corneal wounds are only very obvious if they are large, then they look like fairly distinct rips. Such wounds are very painful and therefore accompanied by restlessness, spasms of the eyelids and much watering of the eye.

● **Pierced cornea**

● If the injury is serious enough, the cornea may be completely pierced.
In this case the eye may appear shrunken; check whether inner parts stick out through the wound, for example the iris which is easily noticed because it is coloured.

TREATMENT

■ If abrasion is suspected, then clean the eye with an eyewash only.
Do not use drops unless advised by the vet. These often contain corticosteroids that are harmful in cases of injury to the cornea.

■ Deep corneal cuts, and above all, perforations are subject to infection and may also cause internal damage to the eye. They therefore require prompt veterinary attention.
In the meantime you can gently clean the eye and, if necessary, bandage it to protect it following the illustrations on pages 110-111.

Foreign bodies in the eye

These are usually located in the conjunctival sac behind the eyelids. Small or pointed bodies can also penetrate the cornea.

CAUSES

★ **Small seeds, fragments of plants or grass awns.** These can become lodged behind the lids. The last-named are particularly bad, as they irritate and tend to run deep into the conjunctive membrane. Small foreign bodies, above all blunt ones, are often dislodged by the eye watering.
★ **Thorns, splinters of wood, metal or other material.** When these come into contact with the cornea, they can then remain stuck (fig. 1).

ASSESSMENT

● **Signs**

● The presence of foreign bodies in the eye is very distressing for the animal. You will notice it is restless, frequently blinks, has the affected eye shut and the eye constantly waters; because of the pain, the animal may rub its eye with its paws.
The signs occur particularly in summer, on or following outdoor trips, especially walks in long grass, and usually indicate the presence of foreign bodies.

● **Examination of eye**

● Carefully examine the eye in a good light (direct sunlight, bright artificial light, torch) holding the animal still as shown in the chapter on restraining on page 31.
– First part the eyelids to make the cornea more readily visible.
– Grasp a small fold of skin near the edge of the eyelid and try gently to lift it away from the eye (fig. 2) to observe the conjunctival sac; do this with both the upper and lower lid.
– Although a delicate operation, the third eyelid can be revealed by carefully pressing down on to the eyeball from on top of the upper eyelid (see p. 108).

● **When the foreign body cannot be found**

● How well such a foreign body can be revealed depends on its site; if it is tucked right away under the lid or behind the third eyelid, it will be difficult to see. If this is the case, call the vet at once.

TREATMENT

■ As the eye is very easily damaged, call a vet at once. Only if the vet is not readily available should you see if the foreign body is in a place where you can remove it yourself.
– Hold the animal very firmly to avoid sudden jerks of the head (see Restraining on p. 31).
– Try to grip the foreign body with tweezers (either flat-ended or rounded), taking care not to hold them at a right angle to the eye (fig. 3).
– Extract the foreign body gently but not too slowly because the pain will upset the animal.
– Clean the eye with a gauze pad moistened with antiseptic solution (e.g. boracic acid).

1. Splinter in the cornea
2. Looking for foreign body
3. Extraction

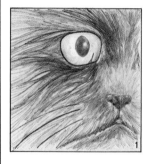

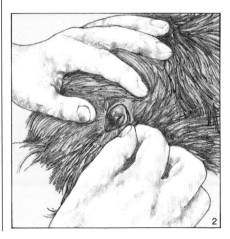

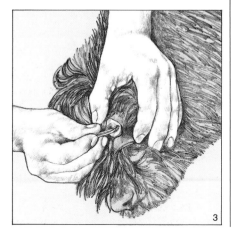

Serious eye injuries

Severe injuries can cause considerable damage, at times beyond repair and leading to blindness.

CAUSES

* **Bruises.** From stones, hard balls etc.
* **Falls from heights.** Often the case with cats and puppies falling from windows and down stairs.
* **Other common causes.** Heavy blows, fights, car accidents.

ASSESSMENT

Serious blows to the eye can cause various types of damage.

● External bleeding

● Bleeding underneath the conjunctiva covering the eyeball will appear as red stains, often quite large around the cornea, in the part of the eye which is normally white (fig. 1).

● Internal bleeding

● The most frequent condition of internal bleeding (i.e. bleeding into the eyeball), mostly involves blood accumulating in front of the lens (see Anatomical diagram on p. 15). It appears externally as a red half-moon beyond the cornea. It can vary in width and will sometimes even obscure the whole pupil (fig. 2).

● Detachment of the lens

● The lens behind the iris (see Anatomical diagram on p. 15) can become detached following injury, and lose its normal position.
You will be able to recognize this condition by the pupillar opening being deformed or becoming opaque (fig. 3).

● Detachment of the eyeball

● In this case the eyeball falls out of its socket. This is a serious injury and is most likely to occur in dogs with a flat face or protruding eyes, such as the Pekingese, and in cats (fig. 4).

• Injury to the cornea and eyelids

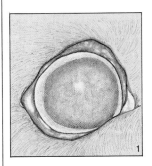

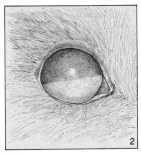

1

2

1. External bleeding
2. Internal bleeding
3. Detachment of the lens
4. Detachment of the eyeball

• These injuries have been dealt with on previous pages: corneal injuries on page 112 and eyelid injuries on page 108.
Other internal eye damage, such as bleeding and detachment of the retina, can be determined only by careful veterinary examination. Even if the animal is not showing any of the signs precisely as they are described here, it may be best to ask the vet to check as soon as possible.

TREATMENT

■ If bleeding from the eye continues, or haemorrhages from the eyelids are apparent, apply cold compresses at once. Fold a piece of gauze several times and dip it in cold water (see p. 109, fig. 2).

■ If the eyeball is out of its socket, make sure that it remains moist and clean by dripping an antiseptic eyewash on to it (e.g. boracic acid or, failing that, clean water or bottled water). This will prevent any further damage caused by the drying of the cornea.

■ Whenever you have to deal with serious injuries to the eyelids or cornea, try to bandage over the wounded eye, following the instructions on pages 110-111. Then consult the vet at once.

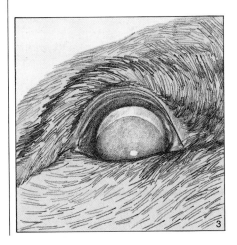

3

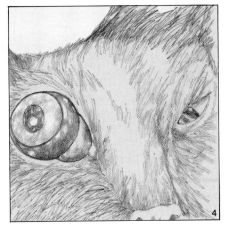

4

EAR INJURIES

Injuries to the ear flap

These injuries are frequent in dogs and cats which are allowed to roam freely.

CAUSES

★ **Bites.** These generally occur during dog fights. They are quite common in tomcats especially during the mating season.
★ **Cuts.** From thorny bushes, barbed wire, broken glass etc.
★ **Gunshot wounds.** Occasionally these will happen to dogs during hunting.

ASSESSMENT

● **Depth of the wound**

● The damage may be superficial, affecting only the outer and inner skin over the ear cartilage; or it

1. Injury to the ear flap of a dog

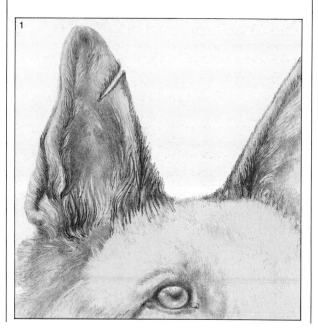

may be deep, in the form of lacerations extending through the whole flap (fig. 1).

● **Extent**

● The degree of injury will vary from case to case, but can involve wounds from a mere scratch to complete severance of part of the flap.

Such wounds are not dangerous but often involve extensive bleeding from broken vessels along the edge of the ear.

Since they tend to heal up leaving an ugly scar, it is best to have them attended to. You should therefore take the animal to a vet as soon as possible.

TREATMENT

■ Stop any bleeding by pressing the edges of the wound between thumb and index finger, to close the cut vessels (fig. 2). After a few minutes let go to check whether the blood flow has stopped. If not, continue to press and, if you have an ice pack handy, cool the part. Bear in mind that bleeding will usually stop, even if it is initially heavy.

2. Treatment of an ear flap injury: stopping the bleeding

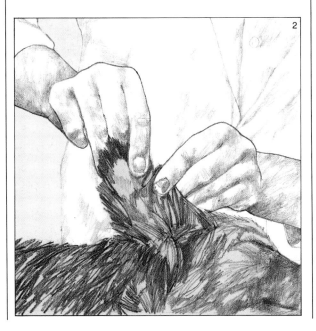

■ Clean the wound with gauze, gently removing any coagulated blood from around its edges together with fragments of hair and other contaminating materials (fig. 1).

If you can, clip the hair surrounding the wound and then disinfect it with a pad soaked in antiseptic solution (non-alcoholic to avoid the stinging upsetting the animal). Hydrogen peroxide or water-based iodine (povidone iodine) or mercurial (merthiolate) solutions are suitable.

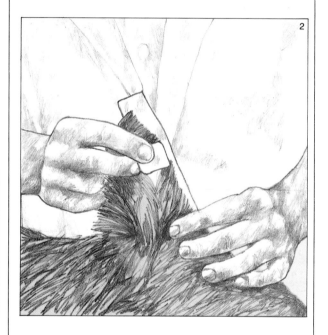

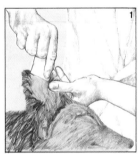

■ Since sudden jerks or shaking of the head can reopen the wound with renewed bleeding, the edge of the flap should have a plaster put on it:

– Put a small pad of gauze over the wound (fig. 2).
– Apply a wide strip of adhesive plaster to the outside of the flap running from the base of the ear to the tip and protruding over the edge by 1–2 cm (½–1 in).
– Put another strip of a similar size on the inside and overlap it with the first strip. They must adhere to the ear and to each other (fig. 3).

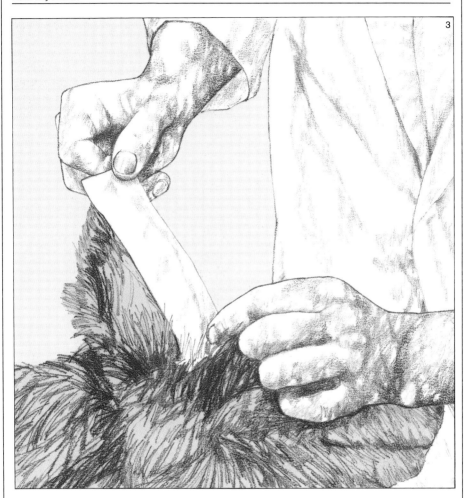

Treatment of an ear flap
injury:
1. Cleaning and disinfecting
2. Protecting with a pad
3. Applying a plaster

Blood blister (haematoma) in ear flap

Blood blisters form as the result of damage to a blood vessel running between the skin and cartilage of the ear. They are more frequent in dogs than in cats, and especially in those with erect ears (e.g. German Shepherd dogs).

CAUSES

★ **Bites.** Common result of fights, particularly in tomcats during the mating season.
★ **Severe shaking of the head.** Blood blisters can be caused by the banging of the flap on nearby objects. You should bear in mind that shaking is often attributable to inflammation of the ear canal (often caused by parasites) or by the presence of a foreign body.

ASSESSMENT

• **Signs**

• A blood blister appears as a plump swelling, soft to the touch, within the wall of the flap and usually towards the tip (fig. 1).
Often, the swelling is not noticed until it is large and the animal is distressed by it, holding the ear low and sometimes shaking it.

The blood flow does not stop quickly and so the swelling tends to grow. Moreover, the blood is reabsorbed only very gradually. The condition disappears very slowly and often leaves the ear distorted ("cauliflower ear").
To prevent this, prompt intervention by the vet is essential. Moreover, you should check for other wounds (see pp. 118–119) and foreign bodies inside the ear (see pp. 126–127).

TREATMENT

■ To reduce the flow of blood, immediately apply a source of cold to the ear (e.g. an ice pack) for at least 10–15 minutes.

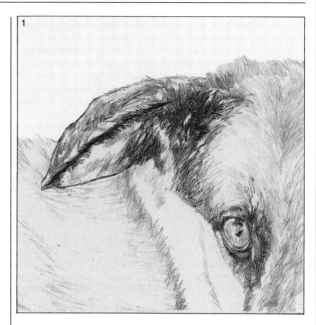

1. Example of a large blood blister in ear flap

■ At the same time press the flap between thumb and index finger below the blood blister to reduce the flow.

■ If prompt veterinary help is not at hand, immobilize the ear to avoid further damage through shaking (see instructions on the next page).

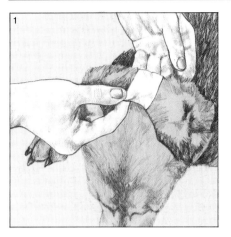

Bandaging the ear

1. The simplest method of immobilizing the ear flap is to put adhesive plaster on the two flaps after folding the affected ear on top of the healthy one; the plaster must not of course touch the blister but pass below it

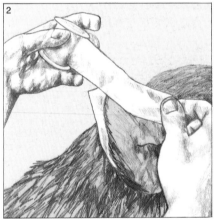

2. Alternatively, immobilize the affected ear only, by putting plaster on its front and back edges, using two strips of adhesive plaster

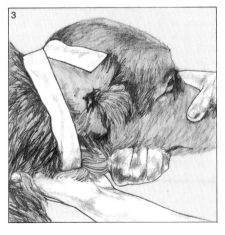

3. One of them should be wound round the neck until it overlaps the piece that is already sticking to the ear

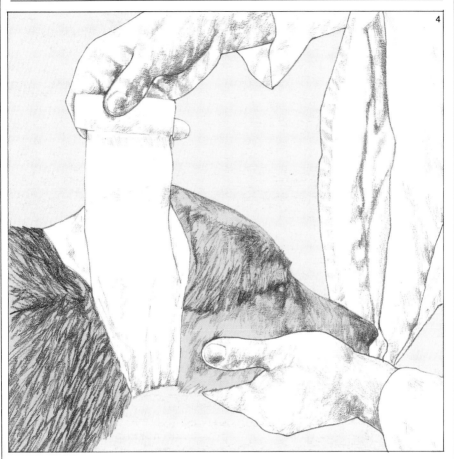

4. Failing plasters of the proper size, bend the ear over the head and fix it in place with gauze bandages or long strips of cloth, winding them round both the neck and the flap. Make sure they are not too tight and will not interfere with breathing

Foreign bodies in the ear

These often occur in dogs, especially those with pendulous ear flaps such as cocker spaniels, but rarely in cats.

CAUSES

★ **Grass awns or fragments.** Grass awns (long-tailed grass seeds) are dangerous because their thin tails and tiny hooks can adhere very easily to the coat. Because of their "barb-like" shape they can only move forwards and are consequently hard to shake off once they are lodged. They may go deep into the ear canal and even injure the ear drum.

★ **Bits of wood and other materials.** These are more easily dislodged by shaking the ears and are therefore less dangerous.

ASSESSMENT

● **Signs**

● If the animal is suddenly restless and shakes its head or holds it on one side and frequently scratches

1. Internal examination of the ear with the aid of a torch

its ear, a foreign body could be lodged in the ear canal, particularly if this occurs during or after a walk in tall dry grass.

● **Examination of the ear**

● Check the ear flap, both inside and out, to exclude the possibility that it may be affected by wounds (see pp. 118-119), blood blisters (see pp. 122-123), ticks and other problems. Then carefully examine the vertical part of the ear canal visible externally, perhaps with the help of an electric torch (fig. 1).
If the foreign body lies further down, seeing and reaching it may be difficult, and a vet must be consulted promptly.

TREATMENT

■ If an awn or other foreign body is found in the outer part of the ear canal, you may be able to extract it with blunt tweezers (fig. 2).
Due to the discomfort, the animal will inevitably move its head around. In order to remove the foreign body effectively, you will have to restrain it appropriately as shown in the chapter on restraining on page 31.

2. Extraction of a foreign body from the ear with tweezers

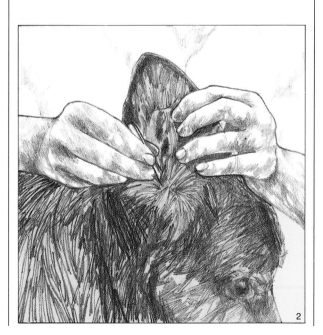

2

NASAL INJURIES

I n animals the nose is very prominent and exposed, so nasal injuries are fairly common both in dogs and cats.

CAUSES

★ **Falls from heights.** Injury to the nose most commonly occurs when dogs and cats fall from heights, from windows and balconies, off roofs and out of trees.

★ **Cuts from sharp objects.** Especially from thorny bushes, barbed wire etc.

★ **Other common causes.** As a result of blows, sustained during fights with other animals or as a result of car accidents.

ASSESSMENT

● **External examination**

● Examine the skin of the nose to see if there are any of the following signs.

Abrasions or tears

Abrasions and tears will usually be easy to see as the hair over the nose of most animals is short and sparse.

Bleeding under the skin

If the injury is severe, it may cause bleeding under the skin.

Damage to bone

Violent blows to the nose may cause varying degrees of damage to the bony structures underneath. In extreme cases, the muzzle can be deformed. The injured part quickly swells.

● **Nosebleed**

● Check whether blood issues from the nostrils (epistaxis) and whether breathing through the nose is impeded.

TREATMENT

■ With bleeding wounds or severe bruises (with or without loss of blood through the nostrils), stop the bleeding and swelling by applying an ice pack, holding it on to the nose for some minutes.

If the part is very painful, apply the source of cold

very gently (fig. 1) and avoid prolonged, forceful pressure on the part which will increase the animal's discomfort.

■ Clean and disinfect the wounds and if there is blood around or within the nostrils, remove it with a gauze pad moistened in a non-alcoholic antiseptic solution (e.g. hydrogen peroxide) until the part is clean.

■ If you find deep wounds and severe damage with heavy bleeding, it will be necessary to consult the vet at once.

1. Application of an ice pack on injured nose

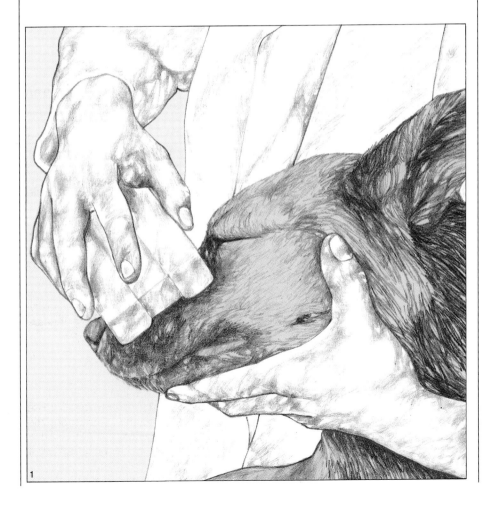

Foreign bodies in the nose

Foreign bodies are sometimes found in the nose, particularly in larger breeds of dogs that have wide nostrils.

CAUSES

★ **Pieces of plant, seeds, small stones.** These foreign bodies are usually breathed in by accident. If they are small and not pointed, they will often come out through sneezing. You will also notice a degree of discomfort because they generally cause increased production of nasal secretions.

★ **Grass awns or fragments.** More dangerous are grass awns or their fragments which, because of their shape, will not come out and are driven further into the nasal cavities.

ASSESSMENT

• **Signs**

• Foreign bodies in the nasal cavities cause much distress and produce repeated sneezing and discharge from the nose. The discharge is generally copious and often involves one nostril only. If these signs are noticed, during or after a walk through tall grass, the presence of a foreign body is suggested.

• **Looking for a foreign body**

• Examine the nostrils with care, using an electric torch with a well focused beam.

Clean away any mucus and try to locate the foreign body. Bear in mind that if it is deep inside, it will not be visible.

1. Extraction of a foreign body from the nose

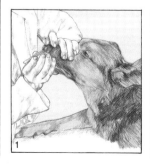

TREATMENT

■ If the foreign body can be easily found, try to remove it by seizing it with tweezers with blunt points. Hold the animal quite still with the aid of a helper (fig. 1). Exercise great care and do not attempt to probe deeply.

If the foreign body cannot be seen, but signs suggest that one is there, a vet must be consulted without delay.

PHYSICALLY CAUSED EMERGENCIES

FROSTBITE

HYPOTHERMIA

HEATSTROKE

BURNS

ELECTRICAL BURNS

FROSTBITE

Frostbite is localized damage caused by intense and prolonged cold, in parts of the body more exposed or less well provided with blood vessels, namely the ears (especially if erect), scrotum, extremities of the limbs, and tail.

CAUSES

★ **Long period of exposure to temperatures below freezing point.** Especially when it is windy and at night.

★ **Prolonged immersion in snow.** Frostbite is a danger when the weather is bad. Animals with short hair are the most susceptible.

ASSESSMENT

* **External examination**

- Check the skin on the points of the ears, the scrotum, tail and the extremities of the limbs; if there is frostbite, this will feel very cold, appear pale and be insensitive to handling.
After thawing, which will occur about 5–10 minutes after being brought into warm surroundings, the skin becomes red, regains its sensitivity, and starts to hurt.

* **Serious frostbite**

- If the tissue is badly damaged, you will notice that the skin gradually peels or, in the most serious cases, even partially detaches. If you observe these developments, you should consult a vet at once.

TREATMENT

■ Wrap the animal in a thick blanket, perhaps warmed beforehand.

■ Carefully warm up the affected parts by gently applying warm water (not over 40°C [104°F]). Paws can be immersed in a small basin; ears, scrotum and tail can be warmed with pads of cloth soaked in warm water for about 10 minutes (fig. 1).

■ When you see the part is beginning to redden as it warms up, dry it gently, and avoid damage by not handling it further.

■ Having warmed up the frozen part, you can apply a thin layer of animal oil (cod-liver oil) or vegetable oil (olive oil, sunflower seed oil) to limit peeling and to soften the skin (fig. 2).

1. Warming the feet with warm water

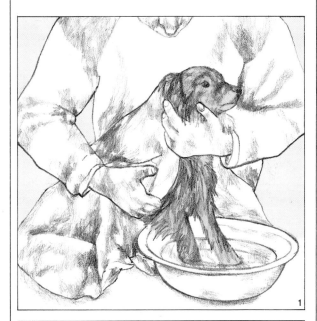

2. Application of oil to soften the skin

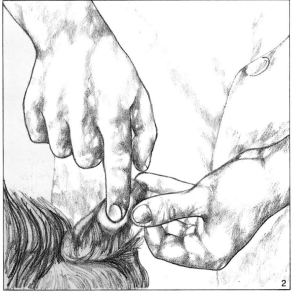

HYPOTHERMIA

Hypothermia *involves cooling of the whole body, internally and externally, and can cause death by slowing down and finally stopping all metabolic functions. The condition is serious but rare, and affects mainly puppies and old and weak animals.*

CAUSES

★ **Long exposure to very low outside temperatures.** This can happen to animals caught in hard weather or without food or shelter, as may happen to animals lost in isolated spots in winter. The risk is increased if the animal does not have a thick coat for protection against the cold.

★ **Accidental immersion in near-freezing water.** Even a few minutes in these conditions can be enough to cause hypothermia.

ASSESSMENT

● **External examination**

● Take the rectal temperature (following the instructions on p. 54) if you have a thermometer available. Check that the heartbeat is not too slow or irregular (see p. 19) and that the animal stays conscious (see p. 101).

If the temperature is below 37°C (98.5°F), the heartbeat slow or erratic, and the animal numb, additional and prompt help is needed from a vet.

1. Sources of heat used to warm up a dog with hypothermia

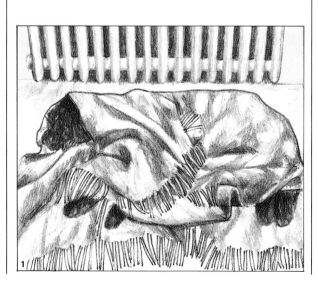

TREATMENT

■ Carry the animal promptly to a warm and sheltered place.

■ If it is wet, dry it with towels, preferably warm ones. Avoid using electric driers as they evaporate the water too fast and can provoke further chilling.

■ Cover the animal with warm woollen blankets and place it in a warm environment (fig. 1). Do not place it in front of any direct heat source because sudden dilation of surface blood vessels can cause withdrawal of blood from internal organs and fatal collapse. Care should be taken to raise the temperature slowly.

■ In case of severe chill, you could put the animal into a warm bath and massage it to reactivate surface circulation. Again, this needs caution.

■ Body temperature tends to rise slowly and unpredictably. Take care to warm the animal slowly and watch for signs of improvement: a more lively appearance; head movements; appearance of shivers and a faster, more regular heartbeat. After about 20 minutes, check the rectal temperature.

2. Using a warm bath to heat a dog with hypothermia

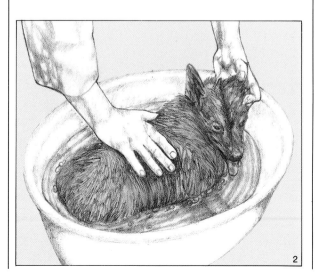

2

HEATSTROKE

Unlike man, cats and dogs do not sweat but eliminate heat in other ways: dogs, by faster and shallower breathing with open mouth to evaporate nasal secretions and extended tongue; cats, by licking, so that saliva on the coat evaporates. If the body temperature rises abnormally high, animals develop heatstroke, especially those kept in very hot and badly ventilated surroundings, which defeat normal heat regulation.

CAUSES

★ **Being kept in cars parked in the the sun.** The most common cause is being kept too long in a car exposed to direct sunlight with the windows closed.

ASSESSMENT

● A rise in body temperature causes a marked increase in the rate of breathing, with the neck and tongue extended, and sometimes a frantic search for openings that might let in some air. Eventually the worsening situation will result in the animal collapsing and finally becoming unconscious. If you have a thermometer, take the rectal temperature (p. 54) which may go beyond 40°C (104–105°F). The heat will be obvious just by putting an open hand on the body or head of the animal.

TREATMENT

■ Carry the animal to a shady and well-ventilated spot.

■ Wet it thoroughly with cold water and fan it with a paper or a piece of cardboard to evaporate the moisture and in consequence lower the temperature. If you have a garden hose handy, use it to gently wet the animal without alarming it. Alternatively, the animal can be immersed in water, keeping its head above water.

■ When it regains consciousness, apply a source of cold, such as an ice pack, to the head and keep it there for several minutes.

■ If you must transport the animal by car, wait for 30 minutes or more before starting the journey; ensure that the interior remains well-ventilated and, if necessary, wet the animal's head and back from time to time.

BURNS

Burns refer to damage to the outer body tissues, from direct contact with high temperatures. Electrical burns and chemical (caustic) ones are dealt with in other chapters.

CAUSES

★ **Contact with boiling water, oil or other liquid.** Accidental scalding when saucepans are upset, or the liquid itself is licked.
★ **Direct contact with flames.** Can occur during fires such as field fires.
★ **Contact with hot metal objects.** The most frequent burns are from irons, saucepans, grills, and hotplates.
★ **Walking over newly tarred roads.** Burns can result when the tar is still hot.

ASSESSMENT

● **Factors determining seriousness**

● In order to assess the seriousness of the burn at the time of the accident, take the following factors into consideration.

Heat source

Burns caused by contact with hot liquid, defined as scalds, and burns from fire, provoke the worst injuries. Boiling oils, being much hotter, are more harmful than boiling water. Contact with steam causes injury to tissues, particularly to the eyes and the outer respiratory passages, since the haircoat gives good protection over the skin. Hot solid objects (mainly metal) cause severe but more localized burns.

Length of contact

The longer the exposure, the more serious the damage will be. It is therefore important to intervene promptly and remove the source of heat instantly.

Size of burned area

If over half the body surface is affected, the burn is usually fatal.

Site of burn

Because of the serious consequences, burns to the head, especially if affecting the eyes and mouth, will result in the worst injuries. Similarly burns near joints are potentially incapacitating, as the scars may later impair mobility.

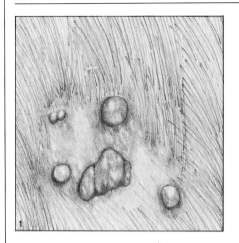
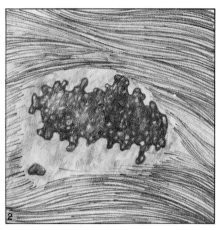

Age and state of health	Young, old or sick animals cannot tolerate the systemic consequences of burns very well.
● **Appearance of burns**	● Burns are classified according to the size and depth of the injury.
First degree burns	In first degree burns there is only a fierce reddening of the skin due to surface blood vessels being dilated by heat. They are the least serious type of burn and will resolve spontaneously in a few days, without leaving any residual signs.
Second degree burns	Second degree burns, in addition to the reddening, are marked by the appearance of blisters due to the accumulation of serum from the damaged surface layers of the skin. This type takes longer to heal because a new skin surface must form. No skin is shed and there is less risk of scars (fig. 1).
Third degree burns	Damage due to third degree burns is such that the complete thickness of the skin and the tissues beneath are destroyed, later drying and forming crusts. Healing is slow and produces conspicuous scars (fig. 2).
● **Systemic effects**	● The appearance of systemic effects, involving the entire body, depends on how serious and extensive the burns are. Since this is a very painful injury, it usually produces shock several minutes later with lowered blood pressure and a loss of sensation, which disappear after a few hours.

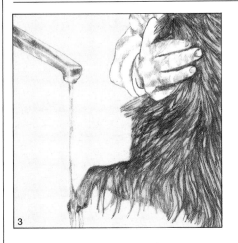 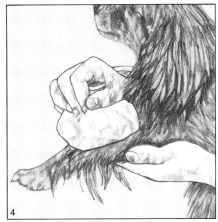

Appearance of burns:
1. Second degree burns
2. Third degree burns

Cooling of burn:
3. With running cold water
4. With an ice pack

With extensive second or third degree burns there is a loss of liquid from the injured area and toxins are formed causing a deterioration in condition, usually two to three days later, which is sometimes fatal.

TREATMENT

■ Immediately cool the injured area with cold running water for several minutes. Paws can be put directly under a tap, and other parts of the body can be continuously sprayed with a shower. It is vital to take action immediately.

■ If available, you can apply an ice pack for 10–15 minutes (fig. 4). Extremities can be immersed in a basin containing water and ice cubes.

■ Dry the part gently by dabbing it and avoid rubbing.

■ Do not apply creams, ointments or oils, just protect the wound; if deep, use gauze (ideally sterile), pieces of cloth or clean handkerchiefs (ideally without creases). Avoid using cotton wool.
If there are any blisters, do not break them.
Extensive burns and severe localized burns (second or third degree) need prompt attention from a vet, for treatment both of the affected site and of shock.

ELECTRICAL BURNS

E lectricity, though rarely the cause of accidents, does present a risk of danger for animals, especially those that live in the house.

CAUSES

★ **Licking or biting electrical plugs, cables or flexes.** Contact with electricity usually results from deliberate interference. Most cases are caused by contact through the mouth. The animals most subject to this risk are puppies and kittens because of their inquisitive nature. Before taking one into the household, take care to cover socket outlets if the holes are exposed, and remove or protect hanging flexes.

ASSESSMENT

● **Factors determining the seriousness**

● The seriousness of the electrical burn depends on the type of current, the intensity, i.e. the voltage, and the length of contact.

Type of current

An alternating current is more dangerous than a direct one. The current used for domestic mains is alternating.

Current and voltage

The higher the voltage and current, the worse the shock will be.

Length of contact

Contact for a short time, even with strong currents and high voltage, need not be fatal, as in the case of electrical shocks. However, muscular spasm caused by the contact may result in contact being unduly prolonged.

● **Injuries**

● Injuries caused by electrical contact look like localized burns at the point of contact and are often deep. Sometimes there is also a burn at the exit point of the current, for example the extremities of the limbs.

● **Systemic effects**

● As a direct consequence of the electricity and the pain from such burns, the animal may enter a state of shock characterized by lowered blood pressure, numbness or even complete loss of consciousness.

The main danger of this type of accident is the cessation of breathing from spasm of the respiratory muscles, the stopping of the heart or an altering of its rhythm.

Check at once heartbeat (see p. 98) and breathing movements (see p. 98). If the burn is serious and if breathing or heart rate are abnormal, you must seek the attention of a vet immediately. If breathing has stopped, begin artificial respiration (see p. 142).

TREATMENT

■ Make sure that electrical contact is broken. If it has not been broken, do not touch the animal but turn the electricity off at the main switch, or try to remove the flex concerned by means of a piece of wood or plastic (fig. 1).

1. Distancing the electrical contact using a stick

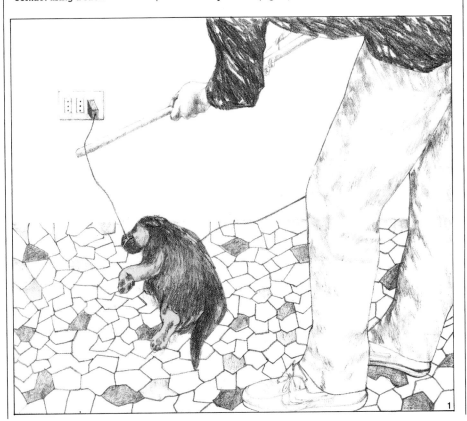

1

Artificial respiration:
1. Correct position for
introducing air into mouth

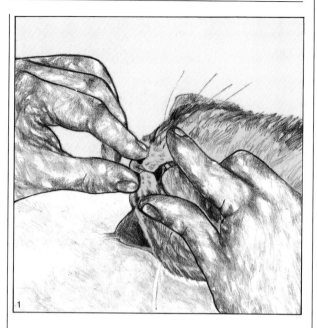

■ Ascertain that there are normal heartbeats, breathing movements and a state of consciousness. If everything is normal, check at once for burns at the point of contact.
Treatment of burns is the same as described on page 139 including prolonged, careful washing with cold water and, if available, applying ice to the injured point for at least 10 minutes. This may not be possible if the burnt part is the tongue. In this case, you should check carefully whether there are symptoms of choking, following the root of the tongue becoming swollen.

■ If you find that, although the heart is beating regularly, the animal shows no signs of breathing normally, you will have to apply artificial respiration immediately.

Artifical respiration

– Keep the animal lying on its side with its neck stretched out and head and nose slightly raised.
– Air can be introduced by blowing through the nostrils holding the mouth shut with one hand (usually more successful in dogs), or through the mouth by keeping the nostrils closed between index

Artificial respiration:
2. Pressure on the chest to let
air out

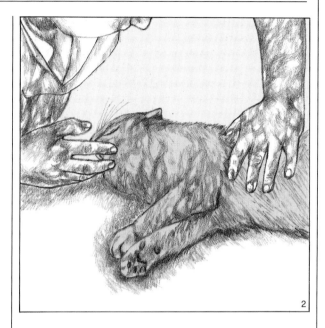

finger and thumb; in this case apply your mouth in front and press lips sideways with one hand to avoid air escaping (fig. 1). The amount of air needed depends on the animal's size. Regulate this by blowing with some force and speed (two to three seconds) until the chest wall rises (i.e. the chest fills) sufficiently.
– Now release the nostrils and press on the chest to let the air out (fig. 2).
Repeat at the rate of 7–10 artificial breathing movements per minute until voluntary breathing reappears.

Cardiac massage

– Sometimes a serious electric shock will stop the heart beating. If this occurs, apply cardiac massage at once to re-start contractions.
– The animal should be positioned lying on its side with neck and head extended to make breathing easier.
– Pass one hand under its chest and place the other directly above it on the other side of the chest, at the point shown (fig. 1 on p. 144).
With cats or small dogs you may need only to apply two or three fingers instead of the whole palm (fig. 2 on p. 144).

– Rapidly compress the chest cavity and repeat rhythmically 60–100 times a minute.
– Continue until the heart beats again and keep checking for some minutes afterwards.

Cardiac massage:
1. On a dog
2. On a cat and small dog

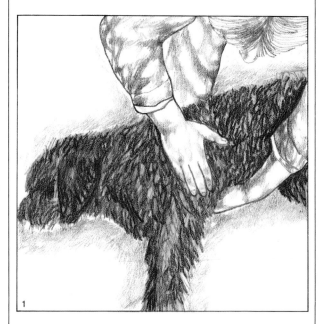

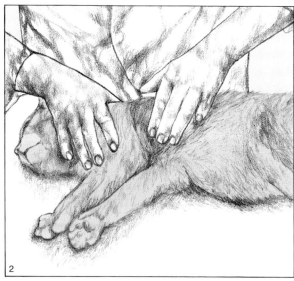

CHEMICALLY CAUSED EMERGENCIES

POISONING

SNAKE BITES

INSECT AND SPIDER BITES

POISONING

Toxic substances or poisons, after entering (or in some cases just being applied to) the body, will cause changes of varying degrees of severity depending on the type and amount taken in. In extreme cases the result can be fatal.

CAUSES

There are various ways in which poisons can be taken in.

★ **Ingestion.** Puppies and kittens tend to lick and eat everything they come across and find interesting. Even in adult dogs, this is the most common way in which they are poisoned.

The process may be direct (often ingestion of plants treated with insecticides) or be an indirect consequence, for example through the ingestion of mice, or moles that have themselves been poisoned.

It can happen that the ingestion occurs involuntarily, as in the case of poisonous substances present on the ground which may be walked through and ingested later when the animal cleans its paws.

★ **Inhalation.** Animals can breathe in poisonous gases, such as carbon monoxide from car exhausts or malfunctioning stoves, or atomized liquids being applied as insecticide treatment.

★ **Direct contact with the skin.** Primarily burns from corrosive substances.

● **Where the effect shows**

How and where the poison will affect the animal can vary. The reaction of the poison may be local, as with caustic substances that cause injury at the point of contact, all over (i.e. systemic) after absorption, or in an organ specifically affected by the poison.

● **Prevention**

The great number of poisonous substances used in the home as well as in industry and agriculture means there are many opportunities for poisoning, especially in animals allowed to roam free. The owner of a pet should be aware of the situations where poisoning could take place, both at home in the house and garden and out on walks, and take care to avoid them. Toxic substances should never be used or left in places where animals wander freely and could be poisoned by them.

On this page there is a list of products in general use which contain toxic substances and could cause poisoning if swallowed. You should take adequate precautions to make sure items such as these are stored out of the way of animals and used under close observation.

On the following pages the tables list the most dangerous and commonly encountered toxic plants and substances, the source of the poisoning and the symptoms of each case.

List of household products that can be poisonous if swallowed

Anti-freeze

Anti-rust solutions

Antiseptics

Bleaches

Coloured pencils

Deodorants

Detergents

   for clothes

   for washing up

   for dishwashers

Dry-cleaning

   preparations

Fire-fighting foams

Fungicides

Glues

Hair dyes

Hair removing creams

Hair sprays

Inks

Insecticides

Matches

Medicated shampoos

Metal polishes

Mothballs

Nail varnish

Paints

Paint and varnish

   removers

Paraffin

Pastel crayons

Perfumes

Petrol

Refrigerants

Rodenticides

Shoe polish

Slug pellets

Soaps

Stain removers

Suntan lotions

Tar

Wax and other

   polishes

Weed-killers

Wood preservatives

TOXIC PLANTS

PLANT	TOXIC PART	TOXIC STRENGTH	SYMPTOMS
Aconitum napellus WOLF'S BANE/ MONK'S BANE	Leaves Seeds Roots	●●	Vomiting, diarrhea Convulsions Death from heart failure
Aquilegia vulgaris COMMON COLUMBINE	Whole plant	●●●	Vomiting, diarrhea Convulsions Death from heart failure
Buxus sempervirens BOX	Leaves	●●	Gastro-intestinal irritation
*Clematis** CLEMATIS	Whole plant	●●	Gastro-intestinal irritation
Colchicum autumnalis COLCHICUM	Whole plant	●●●	Gastro-intestinal irritation Paralysis of muscles and of breathing
Conium maculatum HEMLOCK	Whole plant	●●●	Tremors, convulsions, progressive paralysis Depressed breathing and heartbeat Death

TOXICITY:
- ● moderate
- ●● high, fatal in large doses
- ●●● very high, often fatal
- * all species

TOXIC PLANTS

PLANT		TOXIC PART	TOXIC STRENGTH	SYMPTOMS
	Convallaria majalis **LILY OF THE VALLEY**	Whole plant	●●	Gastro-intestinal irritation Depressed heartbeat
	*Crocus** **CROCUS**	Bulb	●	Gastro-intestinal irritation
	*Delphinium** **DELPHINIUM**	Leaves Seeds	●●	Vomiting, paralysis of limbs Depressed breathing and heartbeat
	*Dieffenbachia** **DIEFFENBACHIA**	Stalk tops	●●	Strong irritation of mouth, gullet, stomach, intestines
	*Euphorbia** **EUPHORBIA**	Whole plant	●	Gastro-intestinal irritation
	Euphorbia pulcherrima **CHRISTMAS DAISY**	Leaves Flowers	●●	Gastro-intestinal irritation
	Galanthus nivalis **SNOWDROP**	Bulb	●	Gastro-intestinal irritation Marked salivation

TOXIC PLANTS

PLANT	TOXIC PART	TOXIC STRENGTH	SYMPTOMS
Gladiolus * GLADIOLUS	Bulb	●	Gastro-intestinal irritation, profuse diarrhea
Hedera helix IVY	Berries Leaves Stalk	●●	Gastro-intestinal irritation In large amounts: depression of nerves and heartbeat
Helleborus Niger HELLEBORE	Whole plant	●●	Strong gastro-intestinal irritation Depressed heartbeat and breathing .
Hyacinthus * HYACINTH	Bulb	●	Gastro-intestinal irritation
Hydrangea macrophylla HYDRANGEA	Leaves Flowers	●●	Stomach pains, vomiting, diarrhea
Ilex aquifolium HOLLY	Berries	●●	Vomiting and profuse diarrhea
Ipomoea purpurea BLUEBELL	Seeds	●●	Hallucinogenic action

TOXIC PLANTS

PLANT		TOXIC PART	TOXIC STRENGTH	SYMPTOMS
	Iris* IRIS	Bulb	●	Intestinal irritation profuse diarrhea
	Lathyrus* SWEET-PEA	Seeds Fruit	●●	Nervous symptoms (paralysis, convulsions)
	Lupinus* LUPIN	Whole plant	●●	Liver disorders Depressed breathing and heartbeat
	Narcissus* NARCISSUS	Bulb	●	Gastro-intestinal irritation Excessive salivation
	Narcissus pseudonarcissus DAFFODIL	Bulb	●	Gastro-intestinal irritation Excessive salivation
	Nerium oleander OLEANDER	Whole Plant	●●●	Gastro-intestinal irritation Depressed nervous system and heart (death from heart failure)
	Parthenocissus quinquefolia CANADIAN VINE	Fruit	●	Gastro-intestinal irritation

TOXIC PLANTS

PLANT		TOXIC PART	TOXIC STRENGTH	SYMPTOMS
	Philodendron * PHILODENDRON	Leaves Stalk	●	Gastro-intestinal irritation In cats: kidney damage
	Ranunculus acer BUTTERCUP	Stalk Lymph	●●	Strong irritation through contact (mouth gullet, stomach, intestines)
	Rhododendron * RHODODENDRON	Leaves Flowers	●●	Vomiting Nervous symptoms
	Taxus baccata YEW	Leaves Seeds	●●●	Gastro-intestinal irritation Tremors, convulsions Collapse of heart and circulation, death
	Tulipa * TULIP	Bulb	●	Gastro-intestinal irritation
	Viscum album MISTLETOE	Berries	●●	Gastro-intestinal irritation Nervous symptoms (unco-ordinated movements) Hyper-salivation
	Wisteria * WISTERIA	Seeds Fruit	●	Gastro-intestinal irritation

THE MOST COMMON POISONS

POISON	SOURCE OF POISONING	SYMPTOMS
ACETONE	Paint solvents	By inhalation: irritation of bronchi and lungs By ingestion: vomiting, diarrhea, depressed breathing and heartbeat
ALPHACHLORALOSE	Rodenticides	Weakness, anaesthetic effect Lowered body temperature
ANILINE (dyes containing aniline)	Coloured pencils Pastel crayons Paints	Vomiting Impaired breathing Convulsions
ANTI-COAGULANT RODENTICIDES	Rodenticides Mole Killers	Spontaneous bleeding, blood in urine and faeces Depression
ANTU (ALPHANAPHTHYL-THIOUREA)	Rodenticides	Vomiting Serious oedema of the lungs Impaired breathing
ARSENIC	Rodenticides Weed-killer Paints Wood preservatives	Vomiting, diarrhea and stomach pains Tremors Cyanosis Collapse of heart and circulation
BARBITURATES	Sleeping pills	Depressed brain function Coma Depressed breathing
BENZENE	Fuels Solvents Detergents	Vomiting Convulsions Collapse
CAMPHOR	Mothballs Medicinal products	Gastro-intestinal irritation Nervous excitation

THE MOST COMMON POISONS

POISON	SOURCE OF POISONING	SYMPTOMS
CARBAMATE	Insecticides Parasiticides	Tremors, unco-ordinated movements, muscular spasms Vomiting
CARBON MONOXIDE	Burning of organic matter in enclosed spaces	Unco-ordinated movements Weakness Impaired breathing
CARBON TETRACHLORIDE	Fire-fighting foams Dry cleaning preparations	Serious damage to liver and kidneys
CYANIDES	Rodenticides Weed-killers	Asphyxia, coma, swift death
ETHYLENE GLYCOL	Anti-freeze	Gastro-intestinal irritation Convulsions Blocked kidneys
FLUORACETATES	Rodenticides	Nervous excitation Muscular spasms Convulsive fits Collapse of heart and circulation
FORMALIN	Domestic and industrial disinfectants	Serious gastro-intestinal irritation Collapse of heart and circulation
HEXACHLOROPHENE	Soaps and antiseptic solutions	Vomiting, diarrhea, stomach pains Liver and nervous disorders
LEAD	Paints, varnishes Fuels	Acute poisoning: gastro-intestinal irritation Nervous symptoms: excitation, progressive paralysis
MERCURY	Fungicides Weed-killers Insecticides Disinfectants	In acute form: serious gastro-intestinal irritation, stomatitis Convulsions and coma
METALDEHYDE	Slug pellets Solid fuel pellets	Nervous symptoms: spasms, tremors and lack of co-ordination

THE MOST COMMON POISONS

POISON	SOURCE OF POISONING	SYMPTOMS
METHYLATED SPIRIT	Solvents Fuels	Vomiting and stomach pains Nervous excitation Convulsions
NAPHTHALENE	Mothballs	Gastro-intestinal irritation Anaemia and jaundice
NITRATES AND NITRITES OF SODIUM AND POTASSIUM	Fertilizers Meat preservatives	Vomiting and diarrhea Loss of balance, tremors Impaired breathing
NITROBENZENE	Shoe polishes and dyes	Vomiting Lack of co-ordination, convulsions Impaired breathing
ORGANOCHLORINES (DDT, Chlordane)	Insecticides Parasiticides	Nervous symptoms: tremors, spasms, convulsions Excessive salivation
ORGANOPHOSPHATES (trichlorfon, ronnel, diazinon, etc.)	Insecticides Parasiticides	Vomiting, diarrhea Running eyes Excessive salivation Tremors, spasms, convulsions
OXALIC ACID	Bleaches and detergents Stain removers	Oral irritation Serious vomiting and diarrhea
PETROL	Fuels	By inhalation: coughing, impaired breathing, depression By ingestion: vomiting, diarrhea, nervous symptoms
PHENOL	Disinfectants	Vomiting, diarrhea Liver disorders
PHOSPHATES OF ZINC AND ALUMINIUM; WHITE PHOSPHORUS	Rodenticides Mole killers	Gastro-intestinal irritation Jaundice, blood in urine Convulsions
QUATERNARY AMMONIUM COMPOUNDS (e.g. benzalkonium chloride)	Detergents Antiseptics	Vomiting and stomach pains Collapse of heart and circulation

THE MOST COMMON POISONS

POISON	SOURCE OF POISONING	SYMPTOMS
ROTENONE	Insecticides Parasiticides	Gastro-intestinal irritation
SOAPS	Washing powders especially dishwasher powders	Gastro-intestinal irritation
SODIUM HYPOCHLORITE	Bleaches Disinfectants	Irritation and burning effects on skin and mucous membranes
SODIUM PERBORATE	Bleaches	Irritation and burning on skin and mucous membranes
SQUILL	Rodenticides	Vomiting, diarrhea Weakness Changes in heart rate
STRONG ACIDS (sulphuric, hydrochloric, nitric etc.)	Cleaning products Metal cleaners Defoliants	Serious burns through contact or ingestion
STRONG ALKALIS (caustic soda, caustic potash, quicklime etc.)	Detergents for metals, crockery and glass	Serious burns through contact or ingestion
STRYCHNINE	Rodenticides	Nervous excitation Violent muscular spasms
TAR AND DERIVATIVES	Tarred roads, roofs and other surfaces Preserved wood	Gastro-intestinal upsets Liver damage
THALLIUM	Rodenticides	Acute poisoning: serious gastro-intestinal irritation Conjunctivitis Nervous symptoms
TRICHLORETHYLENE	Stain removers	Nervous depression Collapse of heart and circulation Liver and kidney damage
TURPENTINE	Paint and varnish removers	Gastro-intestinal irritation Kidney damage, blood in urine Impaired beathing

ASSESSMENT

Diagnosing a case of poisoning is often hard and will need the confirmation of the vet.
If you suspect that an animal has been poisoned by some product or plant, or if it is showing some of the symptoms, try to find out the following:

● **What has been swallowed or inhaled**

● Check whether there are toxic plants in the house or garden, on balconies or terraces and what poisons may have been easily reached (e.g. mothballs in wardrobes, domestic products not safely locked up etc.).
– Try to find out if there has been any herbicide or insecticide sprayed on land, plants or refuse areas.
– Check to see if any bait or rat and mice poisons have been used in cellars, yards and gardens (you can ask gardeners, caretakers and neighbours as well).

If you think you have found a possible source of poisoning, try to discover exactly what sort of poison is involved.

● **What amount has been taken**

● This can sometimes be established by checking what parts of a plant have been ingested, or how much of a mixture is missing, or what the concentration of poison is in a certain product (you should refer to the original container).

● **How long ago it was taken**

● This is often hard to find out, unless the animal is caught in the act. Try at least to establish an approximate time.

The more accurately these questions can be answered, the easier and more efficient the vet's task will be.

TREATMENT

■ If you observe some of the symptoms that can be caused by poisoning, you should consult the vet at once.
It is desirable to help the animal yourself if the poison has just been taken, that is to say in the last half an hour, or if a vet is not available immediately.

■ **Remove the animal from the source of poisoning**

– If the poison has been ingested, make sure no more is taken. After causing vomiting (see below), rinse the animal's mouth out with water to wash out any residues before it swallows them.
– In cases where the animal has inhaled poisonous gases or vapours, carry it promptly into the open air.
– Thoroughly wash with water the parts of the skin that have come in contact with caustic material.

■ **Try to induce vomiting**

■ Measures to induce vomiting should be taken under the following conditions:
– If the poison has been ingested.
– If less than 30 minutes have elapsed since it was taken.
– If the toxic substance has no irritating or caustic effect.
To provoke vomiting the following can be used:
– Concentrated tepid solutions of water and mustard or salt, in amounts depending on the size of the animal.
– A large crystal of washing soda.
If the procedure works, keep the vomit for the vet to examine.

■ **Antidotes**

■ These are drugs with specific actions and will usually be given by a vet.
In cases of external corrosive burns or ingestion, first wash the affected area thoroughly with running water and then use specific solutions according to the poison, either locally, or by persuading the animal to swallow them, for example:
– Water and vinegar or water and lemon juice to neutralize the action of alkalis (caustic soda, potassium hydroxide, quicklime etc.).
– Water and bicarbonate of soda or water and soap (only externally) to neutralize the action of acids (sulphuric etc.).
– If these are not available, use water alone.
Milk is used as an antidote for certain corrosives (e.g. petroleum products) and heavy metal poisoning (lead, mercury etc.).
The fats in milk can favour the intestinal absorption of toxic substances used as insecticides, herbicides, fungicides and other poisons soluble in fat. Indiscriminate use must therefore be avoided, since it may possibly make matters worse.

POISONOUS SNAKE BITES

W hile there are many species of poisonous snakes in America and Asia, the only really dangerous and widespread one in Europe is the adder, also known as viper.

CAUSES

★ **Adder bites.** These are especially common in dogs, usually in summer and during walks in isolated areas.

ASSESSMENT

First try to discover whether the bite is really from an adder. This will not be a problem if you saw the animal being bitten and were able to observe the snake.

Often, however, the attack will happen when the animal is on its own, out of sight. For this reason it is important to know how to recognize the symptoms.

• **Signs of a bite**

• An animal bitten by a snake is usually restless, shaking and licking the injured spot; dogs may howl with pain and fright.

Carefully examine the area where you think it was bitten and look for the two fang marks. These are usually about 1 cm (½ in) apart and have a dark red edge to them (fig. 1 on next page). The wound will swell up quite quickly and often to a considerable size.

• **Signs of poisoning**

• The systemic signs of poisoning are gradually increasing weakness, sometimes vomiting and a marked thirst. In the final stages impaired heart rate and breathing develop which can subsequently lead to death.

The speed with which these signs appear (from a few minutes to a few hours) and their severity depend on how much poison was injected and whereabouts in relation to the density of blood vessels in the area, as well as how soon you intervened.

TREATMENT

■ Locate the wound made by the bite and make it bleed at once to wash out some of the poison. Apply some pressure with your finger around the bite. If this does not cause enough blood to flow, use the point of a sharpened knife blade to make an incision for each fang mark (fig. 2).

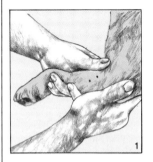 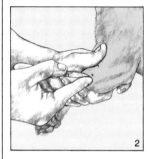 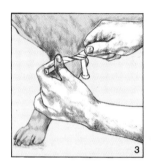

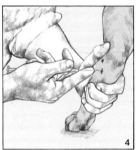

Do not resort to sucking the blood from the bite if at all possible.

■ With bites on the legs apply a tourniquet above the bite on the body side (fig. 3), to limit the spread of poison in the circulation. Make sure it is not tied so tightly that it could stop the blood flow from the incision.

■ Even though bleeding and stopping the spread of poison are crucial measures, the only really effective remedy is the injection of the appropriate anti-venon.

Many veterinary surgeons hold supplies, especially in the areas where bites are encountered most frequently.

Beware of areas and conditions where snakes may be (basking in the sun, on heaths and moorlands) and keep to recognized paths.

■ Having completed the steps described, organize swift transportation to the nearest vet. The animal must be kept still and quiet, and wrapped in a warm blanket.

The anti-venon is generally injected half around the bite marks and half intramuscularly (fig. 4).

Treatment of an adder bite:
1. Appearance of bite
2. Fang marks
3. Application of tourniquet
4. Injection of anti-venon

Adder: distribution and morphological characteristics

The map shows the distribution in Europe of the most common species of adder

Vipera ammodytes
(Nose-horned viper)
Vipera aspis
(Asp viper)
Vipera berus
(Common viper)
Vipera Latastia
(Lataste's viper)
Vipera seoanei
(Seoane's viper)
Vipera ursinii
(Orsini's viper)

The drawings illustrate:
a) an asp viper
b) detail of head

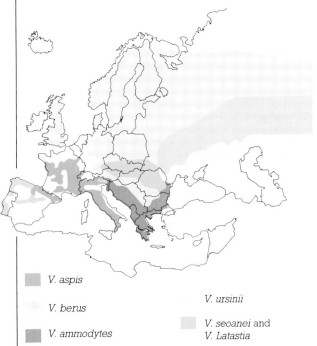

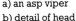 *V. aspis*

V. berus

V. ammodytes

V. ursinii

V. seoanei and
V. Latastia

Adders (or vipers) are medium-sized snakes (40–80 cm [15–30 in]) with a stocky body, a short tail and a head fairly distinct from the neck. The top of the head is covered by scales of irregular size and shape; the eye is medium-sized, with a vertical pupil. The adder's colour varies greatly, depending on its habitat. The spinal stripe is always well-marked and consists of a set of patterns different in the various species and sub-species. The poison fangs fed by two glands, one on each side, are situated at the front of the mouth. When they are at rest they are folded back and are only extended when the snake assumes the attack position with mouth wide open. The common European viper (*Vipera berus*) is the only one found in Great Britain. The markings vary but it usually has a long zigzag down the back with a double row of dark spots to the sides. It will strike quite readily and the bite needs immediate attention.

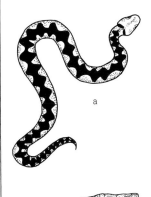

a

b

INSECT AND SPIDER BITES

Insects (bees, wasps, hornets, caterpillars,) and also spiders and scorpions can inject poisons, which will cause local injury and at times systemic effects.

CAUSES

★ **Bees, wasps and hornets.** Stings are frequent in summer and in the vicinity of nests.
★ **Spiders and scorpions.** These can be a problem in hot countries in isolated areas.
★ **Caterpillars.** Rare; in hot climates.

ASSESSMENT

● **Signs**

● Immediately after an animal has been stung by an insect, spider or scorpion, it becomes restless and licks the injured area. The site generally swells conspicuously and therefore it is easy to find. If you part the hair and carefully examine the skin of the swollen area, you can often find the tell-tale bite or sting marks in the center.
You will need to call a vet at once in the following cases:
– When the animal has been stung by a scorpion or has multiple stings from a number of bees, wasps or hornets.
– When there is pronounced and extensive swelling with fever and depression.
– When the sting or bite is in a critical region, such as around the eyes, or in the mouth or throat because the effects could be dangerous, especially if breathing is impaired.

TREATMENT

■ Immediately after the injury, it may help to apply a pad of cotton wool saturated with diluted ammonia (use 1 tablespoonful in 175 ml/6 fl oz warm water). Avoid applying any near the eyes, nose and mouth and check that, when using it, the skin does not become inflamed. Cold compresses could be used but are less soothing. Anti-inflammatory creams or lotions are more effective.

Opposite: illustrations and a brief description of the species that most commonly give unpleasant bites

Bee, wasp and hornet stings

The most common species of insects to give animals painful stings are bees, wasps and, in particular, hornets. They produce, in the glands attached to their sting, a poison containing various toxic substances which cause swellings that at first itch and then hurt. Danger usually arises only if there are many stings (some hundreds from bees or wasps, a few dozen from hornets). This may happen if the animal is attacked by a swarm. Also if the animal is stung in the mouth, it might involve the tongue

Hornet

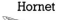

Bee 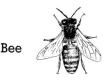 **Wasp**

Caterpillar

swelling and blocking the airway. This could lead to anaphylactic shock and sudden collapse.

Scorpions, spiders and caterpillars found in the hotter regions of the world can inflict painful and sometimes serious stings on animals.

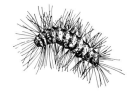

Some species of caterpillars, which have fairly long and sharp hairs on their surface, can provoke inflammatory reactions that cause itching, redness and sometimes blisters or swellings. The irritation is produced by the implanting of minute stings containing poison.

Spider

Some spiders, when provoked, will give a nasty bite. Many produce strong irritants causing local swellings that are hard and painful. Minor cases result in itchy spots. Some rare species produce powerful poisons that act not only locally at the site of the bite but on the whole body, sometimes with fatal results (e.g. the black widow [*Latrodectes tredecimguttatus*] and the tarantula [*Lycosa tarantula*]).

Scorpion

Scorpions inject poison by means of a sting on the end of their tails. The most dangerous species are tropical, but some in temperate zones, though rarely lethal, can produce problems. The injection produces local swelling and in serious cases fever, muscular spasms and impaired breathing and circulation.

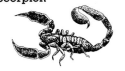

DIGESTIVE
EMERGENCIES

MOUTH INJURIES

FOREIGN BODIES

ABDOMINAL PAIN

ENLARGED AND TWISTED STOMACH

MOUTH INJURIES

M outh injuries in cats and dogs are one of the most frequent types of case requiring first aid.

CAUSES

★ **Serious injuries.** Caused by accidents and, especially in cats, falls from a height.
★ **Chemical burns.** As a result of ingestion, or simply licking at poisonous products, direct contact of them with the skin, or after snake, spider and scorpion bites.
★ **Electrical burns.**
★ **Other common causes.** Fights with other animals or severe blows.

ASSESSMENT

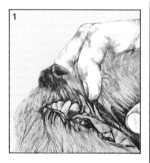

1. A broken canine tooth

First of all examine the lips, to see if there are any bruises or deep wounds, which tend to bleed profusely.
Gently lift the lips and check the upper and lower rows of teeth; broken teeth (fig. 1) are conspicuous, and often occur, especially with damage to the canines. Examine also whether teeth are positioned normally, since they may be displaced even if they are not actually broken.
Slowly and carefully open the mouth and check that this can be done without provoking pain; if the animal shows signs of discomfort, the jaw bone or its joint(s) may be damaged.
Examine the hard palate (the roof of the mouth), which in cases of serious injury, especially in cats, may have split in the middle, and the tongue, which may be lacerated.

TREATMENT

■ Disinfect lip wounds with a non-alcoholic antiseptic and stop any bleeding by pressing a pad of gauze on to the wound site for some minutes. Fractures and dislocations of the teeth and of the jaw, and injuries to the lips and tongue that will clearly require stitching, must receive prompt attention from a vet.

FOREIGN BODIES

Dogs and cats often swallow foreign bodies. Puppies, in particular, will instinctively lick at and swallow objects indiscriminately, either from greed or playfulness. The foreign body may pass through the whole digestive tract and be eliminated with the faeces, or may lodge at some point between the mouth and anus.

CAUSES

★ **Sizeable foreign bodies.** Stones, rubber balls, screws, fruit stones and bottle tops are the type of object that may cause obstructions.

★ **Sharp or cutting foreign bodies.** Nails, needles, pins, fish hooks, wood splinters, fragments of bone, glass and hard plastic can penetrate the mucous membrane lining of the digestive system and may even completely perforate its wall.

★ **Sponges, pieces of cloth, lengths of string, cotton thread or fishing line, with or without needle or hook.** These can all obstruct the intestines.

ASSESSMENT

The signs of a foreign body in the digestive canal will vary according to its location (fig. 3).

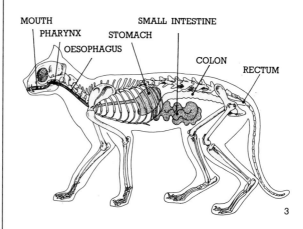

MOUTH
PHARYNX
OESOPHAGUS
STOMACH
SMALL INTESTINE
COLON
RECTUM

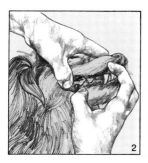

● **Mouth**

2. Examining for foreign bodies in the mouth
3. Position of foreign bodies in the digestive canal

● If the foreign body is in the mouth, the animal is restless and rubs at its mouth with its front paws or rubs its mouth on the ground, swallowing nervously and dribbling saliva.
Raise the lips and check the teeth, to see whether pieces of wood, bone or some other material are stuck there (fig. 2).

Next check the tongue. Gently open the mouth and move the tongue sideways out of the mouth with your fingers to see whether anything has become wound round it, such as bits of string, wire, rubber bands etc., (fig. 1) or stuck into it.
With the help of a torch, examine the inner parts of the mouth.

● **Pharynx and oesophagus**

● If a fairly large foreign body gets stuck in the pharynx, it can seriously impede breathing (see p. 175).
If the foreign body stops in the oesophagus and penetrates the wall or obstructs the passage of food, it is very troublesome and hurts, provoking constant swallowing and pain with much slobbering of saliva that may contain traces of blood if the wall is damaged. If the animal swallows water or food, it usually regurgitates them .
Inspect the back of the mouth with a torch having opened it wide so you can see as far as possible (see fig. 1 on p. 176). It is usually possible to see foreign bodies in the pharynx, though often a vet is needed to identify and remove them. This will certainly be the case if they are further down in the oesophagus.

● **Stomach**

● The main sign of a foreign body stuck in the stomach is vomiting, though it may only be froth that is returned. Attempts at vomiting may recur continually, at frequencies that depend on the type of foreign body and the irritation it causes. Pointed and cutting objects such as slivers of glass are particularly dangerous, whereas smooth foreign bodies may produce few if any signs initially. Check whether the vomited material contains blood.

● **Small intestine**

● Obstruction by a foreign body may provoke frequent attempts at vomiting, often accompanied initially by diarrhea. The abdominal wall can be tense, because of abdominal pain; often there is a fever as well.

● **Colon and rectum**

● The colon and rectum in most cases are obstructed by fragments of bone or wood, and sometimes also by pieces of cloth or plastic. These then mix with the faeces (motions) and form large hard masses. Signs are frequent unsuccessful attempts at defecation, often painful, with the possible passage of mucus, at times tinged or striped with blood.

TREATMENT

If the foreign body is in the mouth, try to extract it (for instance, with a pair of pliers), if this is not too difficult or risky.
In all other cases of the signs described here when a foreign body has been swallowed or you suspect the presence of one, you should promptly consult a vet.

1. Cotton wrapped round a cat's tongue

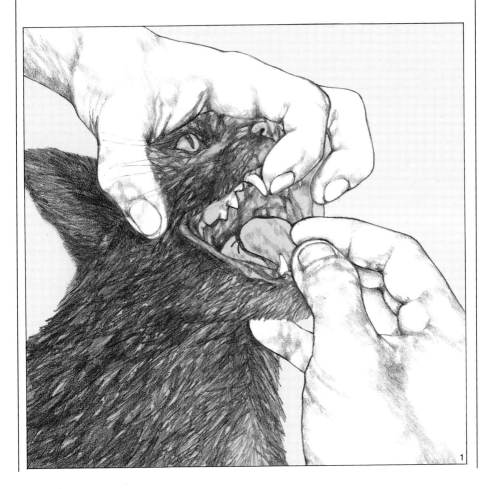

ABDOMINAL PAIN

S evere abdominal pain, often of sudden onset, occasionally affects cats and dogs.

CAUSES

★ **Intestinal spasms.** Usually due to the presence of foreign bodies (see p. 167).
★ **Injuries to abdomen.** When internal organs are damaged.
★ **Poisoning.** Especially those that seriously irritate the stomach and intestine (see table of most common poisons on p. 153).
★ **Acute inflammation.** Peritonitis or pancreatitis.
★ **Other causes.** Various, and may involve other organs apart from the digestive canal such as the kidneys, bladder and liver.

ASSESSMENT

● **Signs**

● Animals with abdominal pain may appear weak and distressed. They assume abnormal positions and are often unable to rise on their hind legs. Vomiting or diarrhea may be present, and breathing is often rapid and shallow.
Gently palpate the abdomen, which you will find is held tense in such cases, and see whether this produces a painful reaction.
Then check the temperature as described on page 54; with certain conditions it will be raised.
Try to find out if the animal may have ingested a foreign body or poison, and ascertain how much food, and of what type, the animal has eaten in its last few meals.

TREATMENT

■ When you notice these signs of abdominal pain, you will need to call a vet promptly who can establish the likely cause and institute appropriate measures.
In the meantime, if the animal is outdoors, put it in a sheltered spot and cover it with a thick blanket if the weather is cold. Transport it gently, avoiding any movement that may provoke pain.

ENLARGED AND TWISTED STOMACH

The stomach can become abnormally dilated due to the formation of gas. This may occur from time to time in large dogs. Twisting of the stomach is serious and turns the dilated stomach on its own axis, thus closing its two openings (cardia and pylorus) and preventing the escape of the gas.

CAUSES

★ **Excessive intake of air, food or water.** Dilatation can occur with the overeating of indigestible or fermentable foodstuffs (bones, bread, cereal etc.) which cause gas production, or the intake of large quantities of air or water which can happen with hasty swallowing. Dilatation at times leads to twisting of the stomach (volvulus).

★ **Rough movements: jumping, rolling or falling.** Movement causing sudden displacement of abdominal organs may, although seldom, also provoke twisting of the stomach.

ASSESSMENT

● An animal with a distended stomach is usually distressed and in pain, often tries to vomit (though this is not possible with twisting) and shows fast, shallow breathing. Examine the abdomen to see if it is increased in size.

If you tap the left side of the abdomen with a finger tip, you may produce a hollow sound because of gas in the distended stomach but vigorous palpation could increase pain and shock, so be gentle and do not persist.

It is hard to know for certain whether twisting has occurred, though this usually results in severe shock and depression.

TREATMENT

■ Cases of dilatation, especially when it occurs to large dogs, will require prompt veterinary attention.

The animal must be transported with the utmost care, avoiding sudden movements. If it is very distressed and in pain, you should arrange to move it as explained on page 106.

BREATHING
EMERGENCIES

DROWNING

FOREIGN BODIES

DROWNING

C ases of drowning are rare in cats and dogs, as these animals are generally good swimmers. It does sometimes happen to puppies, old and sick animals, or those which have been injured and fallen into the water or hurt while swimming.

CAUSES

★ **Drowning in the sea.** Falls from gangways and landing stages, and especially in rough water.
★ **Drownings in lakes, ponds, or rivers.** Particularly those with eddies or strong currrents.
★ **Swimming baths and locks.** These are potentially dangerous because once the animal has fallen or jumped in, it will need help to get out. Otherwise it is likely to drown when it becomes exhausted.

ASSESSMENT

● Once the animal has been taken out of the water, check whether it shows any movement. If the animal seems completely motionless see whether it is still alive by checking for a heartbeat (see p. 98) and breathing. If it is still breathing, you may find it will cough heavily and breathe in and out with difficulty.

TREATMENT

■ Act quickly and try to remove the water from the lungs.
The animal should ideally be held upside down; raise it by its hind legs and hold it around the thighs. Then let the water drain out (fig. 1). Heavy dogs, which are hard to lift up, may be held on their side with their head lower than their chest, for example by hanging them over the edge of a step or a table.
If normal breathing movements are absent, repeatedly apply manual pressure to one or both sides of the chest for a few seconds at a time, to reduce the lung volume and force the water out of the throat.
If, after removal of most of the water, there are no signs of the animal resuming normal breathing, you must resort to artificial respiration as explained on page 142.

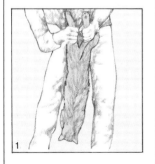

1. How to hold a cat in order to remove water from the lungs

BREATHING OBSTRUCTED BY FOREIGN BODIES

The main cause of choking in cats and dogs is an ingested foreign body blocking the airway. Foreign bodies may lodge at various points (fig. 2). They will stop in the pharynx if they are too big for swallowing. Smaller ones may enter the larynx (voice box), going as far down as the windpipe and bronchi.

CAUSES

★ **Large objects.** Stones, rubber balls, bottle tops and other large round objects are the most likely to obstruct.

★ **Ears of corn.** Also, more rarely, bits of wood or bone can pass into the larynx, windpipe or bronchi and, although they need not completely obstruct the passage of air, they will make breathing difficult.

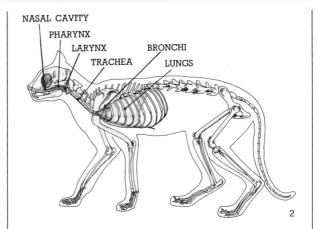

NASAL CAVITY
PHARYNX
LARYNX
TRACHEA
BRONCHI
LUNGS

2

ASSESSMENT

● **Signs**

● If the pharynx or larynx is obstructed by an object that almost completely blocks the passage of air, it will produce choking. In this condition breathing is very difficult and the animal will extend its neck and open its mouth in order to breathe more easily.

If the mucous membranes turn blue or the animal becomes unconscious, the situation is very serious.

Foreign bodies lodged in the windpipe or bronchi usually produce repeated forceful coughing or recurrent choking.

2. Foreign bodies in the respiratory system

1. How to detect a foreign body in the pharynx

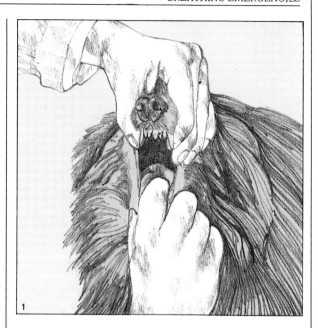

• **Examination of the oral cavity**

• You may be able to see foreign bodies in the pharynx if the mouth is opened wide and the tongue pulled forward as in figure 1. It is a good idea to do this near a good source of light or to shine a torch into the mouth.

TREATMENT

■ If the animal is finding breathing really difficult, it is important to intervene at once.
If the object has been located in the pharynx and can be seen at the back of the mouth, try to remove it with your fingers.
If this fails or if you cannot see the foreign body, seek help to suspend the animal head down, holding it by the hind legs, and slap the side of the chest with your hand (fig. 2). Often this will dislodge the foreign body.
If this move fails, repeat the procedure and, if necessary, compress the two sides of the chest rapidly by hand simultaneously.
Try to avoid causing undue distress to the animal, and always call a vet at once.

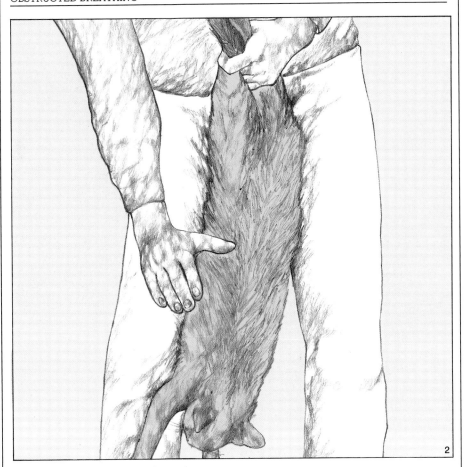

2. How to remove a foreign
body in the respiratory
system

NEUROLOGICAL
EMERGENCIES

PARALYSIS

CONVULSIONS

PARALYSIS

L *oss of the power to move is due to interference with the nerves controlling muscles.*

CAUSES

★ **Serious injuries** (see p. 98). If the animal is seriously injured, the skull, spinal column, pelvis or limbs may be affected in such a way that the nerves and nerve centers that determine movement are damaged.

★ **Hernia or intervertebral discs.** These discs link and articulate the vertebrae. The inner part of a disc may protude and compress the adjacent spinal cord, impeding the transmission of impulses in the nerve fibers as a result.

Sudden hind limb paralysis occurs especially in basset hounds, dachshunds, Pekingese, beagles, cocker spaniels and cross-bred dogs with short legs and a long body.

ASSESSMENT

External inspection may be enough to see where and how severe the problem is. Radiography may be desirable later.

● **Site**

● Paralysis of a single limb is usually due to damaged peripheral nerves; if both hind legs are affected, the spinal cord is injured in the chest, or more usually, in the lumbar regions (see Anatomical diagram on p. 10); if all four legs are involved, the neck or skull is damaged.

● **Severity**

● To assess the severity, you should take into consideration the animal's mobility, muscle tone, the sensitivity of its limbs, and briefly examine the spine.

● **Mobility**

● Check whether the limbs retain some ability to move. In less serious cases the animals still have some degree of movement, though without co-ordination. In more serious cases the limbs are completely paralyzed.

● **Muscle tone**

● Paralysis due to injury to the limbs or the lowest

part of the spinal column (affecting hind legs only) decreases muscle tone and muscles appear limp. If damage occurs in the thoracic part of the spinal column or in the anterior part of the lumbar region, the muscles of the hind limbs increase in tone and the limbs appear rigid and are extended (spastic paralysis).

● **Sensitivity**

● The sensitivity of the skin can be tested by pinching the skin of the limbs at several points to provoke a pain reaction in the animal: if it can feel it, it will react by turning, whining or miaowing, or trying to move away. The same procedure performed on the skin between the toes may cause the foot to be drawn away (pedal reflex, see p. 103). However this alone, without the animal turning or reacting similarly, does not show that the animal is aware of what is happening or is capable of any conscious voluntary movement, but only that the involuntary mechanism (reflex arc), which depends upon the nerve centers in the spinal cord and the associated nerves, is intact.

Lack of conscious sensitivity in the paralyzed area implies severe injury.

● **Examining the spinal column**

A gentle examination of the spinal column might detect conspicuous deviations of the spine and identify the point of injury by observing reaction to pain (see p. 103). If there is possible severe injury, do no persist but consult a vet immediately.

A case of partial paralysis is called paresis. Other forms are distinguished by the area affected: a single limb; legs only; all four limbs; or the limbs of one side.

A true emergency situation is present only if paralysis arises suddenly.

TREATMENT

■ The only way to ensure a correct diagnosis and effective treatment in these cases is to call a vet. You should follow the recommended ways of moving the animal as described on page 106.

CONVULSIONS

Convulsions are a series of rapid and repeated muscular contractions of sudden onset, usually transient. They are often accompanied by loss of consciousness. Although they are also called epileptic fits, in practice this term refers to a specific brain disorder (true epilepsy).

CAUSES

There are many different conditions that can cause an attack of convulsions. The following are some of the principal and most frequently encountered ones:

★ **Hypoglycaemia.** Here convulsions are due to a marked fall in blood sugar to an abnormally low level. They can be the result of serious metabolic disorders, though they may also occur in hounds or working dogs during hard work.

★ **Calcium deficiency.** Convulsions may follow giving birth during the early part of lactation (see p. 136).

★ **Heatstroke.** As well as loss of consciousness, this can cause convulsions (see p. 136).

★ **Damage to the brain.** This can affect the heart or lungs and temporarily diminish blood supply and oxygen to the brain, resulting in fainting and sometimes convulsions.

★ **Poisoning.**
See table of the most common poisons on page 153.

★ **Skull injuries.**
For these cases see page 100.

★ **Kidney or liver disease or inflammation of the brain.** Mainly viral (e.g. canine distemper).

★ **Brain tumours.**

★ **True (or primary) epilepsy.** Characterized by bouts of convulsions not due to any specific cause. It occurs more often in dogs, and mainly in poodles, cocker spaniels, Irish setters and St. Bernards, although it is not unknown in any breed or cross-bred dog.

ASSESSMENT

● **Signs**

● Convulsive attacks usually come on suddenly. True epileptic fits may be preceded by a phase known as an aura, characterized by a state of fear and bewilderment.
Animals in convulsion are often unconscious and lie

on their side. First, the limbs may be stretched out in a strong contraction of several seconds. Then, they begin to move in rhythmic spasms or disjointed jerks. The animals often salivates profusely and urinates and defecates involuntarily.

● **Length of attack**

● An attack of convulsions will generally last a few minutes. The animal will then become conscious but remain disorientated and confused for a time lasting from several minutes to, exceptionally, several hours.

It is important to observe carefully how the "attack" develops, noting how long it lasts, so you can report the findings to the vet.

Repeated convulsive attacks recurring at short intervals, or those that seem not to stop and last over 15 minutes, threaten the animal's life and must be promptly treated by a vet.

● **Other useful information**

● It is also useful to tell the vet what the dog was doing beforehand, what and how much food it last had and when. Also, try to remember any possible injuries during previous weeks, and inform him of any diseases currently present or from which the animal has just recovered.

TREATMENT

■ The only time you can really effectively help the animal is when the attack is due to heatstroke (see p. 136).

■ However, certain measures should be observed in any case of convulsions to ensure the animal's health is not jeopardized any further.

– Do not move the animal during the attack, unless it is in a dangerous position.
– Do not try to open its mouth or prevent its movements.
– Remove any objects that the convulsing animal might knock into and break, causing itself an injury as a consequence.
– Dim bright lights and shut off sources of noise such as radios, televisions, record players and electrical equipment.

OBSTETRICAL EMERGENCIES

GIVING BIRTH

POST-PARTUM PHASE

GIVING BIRTH

Difficulties in reproduction generally occur at the time of giving birth and immediately afterwards.

It helps to be informed on the various stages of reproduction, from mating to lactation, in order to spot serious trouble as soon as it arises. You can then assess how grave it is and tell the vet, whose help thus becomes more effective.

Sexual cycles, pregnancy and the stages of labour are all dealt with in the chapter on reproduction on page 208.

ABNORMAL CONDITIONS

Occasionally abnormalities may occur during birth, both in cats and dogs. It is important to be able to recognize these.

● **Pregnancy lasting too long**

● A pregnancy that greatly exceeds the normal length suggests that the foetuses may be dead. Check for possible unpleasant vaginal discharges (these are generally dark and foul smelling) and observe the animal's general demeanour. Alertness and appetite are always diminished in such cases due to toxins.

● **Uterine inertia**

● This is characterized by weak, or no contractions. It may be present soon after the start or develop after some of the young have been expelled.

With this condition no obvious pushing occurs. If there are contractions, they are weak. Expulsion of the foetuses may occur, but very slowly.

● **Unproductive straining**

● If after two hours no young have been born, their passage may be impeded in the birth canal. The causes can be in the mother (for example an abnormally narrow pelvic canal following pelvic fracture) or in the young animal (too big, in an abnormal position, or two present in the birth canal at once). In such cases, after several attempts straining becomes gradually weaker.

● **Intervals are too long**

● If the interval between the birth of one young animal and the next is too long, it may be due to the uterus becoming tired or be an indication of a difficult birth ahead.

If this is the case, check whether there appear to be young still inside to establish whether parturition is completed or not.

However, bear in mind that in normal circumstances there can be one interval of up to 24 hours (in cats 48 hours) between expelling each of the young.

• Abnormal presentation

• Sometimes the young animal is badly positioned during birth. This will mean the mother will have difficulty in expelling it.

– A shoulder presentation shows only one foreleg, while the other and the head are folded back inside.
– A breech presentation shows the tail only, while the hind legs are folded foward.
– In a neck presentation the head is bent forward and prevents the animal from coming out.

• Possible intervention

• If any of the above cases arises during birth in a cat or dog, you should call the vet at once.

Effective help from you is possible only if during expulsion of a normally positioned kitten or puppy (head, neck and both forelegs, or tail and hind legs, already outside) the pushing is insufficient for complete expulsion.

In that case, pull at the same time that the female pushes, exerting only gentle force so as not to injure the young.

Secure the young animal between thumb and index finger at the base of the skull, at the hips or at the root of the tail, depending on the type of presentation. It is advisable to avoid grasping only the limbs.

Traction may be improved holding the young animal through a towel, and birth may be facilitated by lubricating the young near the vulva with a little vegetable oil or "Vaseline."

If a newly born animal remains attached by the umbilical cord to the placenta still inside, and the mother cannot quickly eliminate the placenta by further straining, help her by tearing (not cutting) the cord about 5 cm (2 in) away from the young animal's body.

THE POST-PARTUM PHASE

I n the post-partum phase certain emergency situations may arise concerning the puppies' or kittens' health, the production of milk and the involution of the uterus.

THE YOUNG

When puppies and kittens are born, they usually receive all the maternal care they need. First, they are licked clean of the amniotic fluid that covers them and which may still block the mouth and nose.
The foetal membranes are chewed and ingested, and the umbilical cord is cut. The mother makes sure the young are near her, to keep them warm and start them suckling.

• If maternal care is lacking

• Sometimes the mother, if nervous or inexperienced, partly or wholly neglects the young, waiting until parturition is complete before paying them any attention, if at all. If this is the case, you should take certain measures.

1. Drying a newborn puppy with a cloth

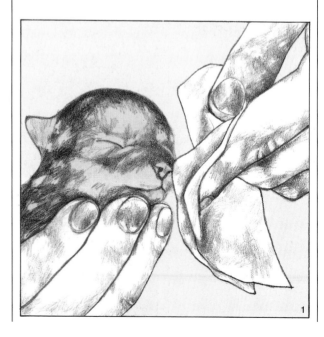

– Remove the foetal membrane, if it is still present over the animal, by tearing it. Do not cut it with scissors or blades, only use your hands, having carefully washed them.
– Dry the young with a clean cloth, warming it beforehand if possible.
Above all, you should clean around the nose and mouth (fig. 1).
– Cut the umbilical cord 5 cm (2 in) from the abdomen, with a pair of large sharp scissors that have been washed and disinfected (fig. 2). Or you can tear it with your fingers, having washed them thoroughly, by squeezing it strongly between thumb and index of both hands and stretching it. This second method reduces bleeding but requires a certain degree of confidence and expertise.
– Try putting the young near the mother. If that disturbs her or leaves her indifferent, keep the young clean and warm but apart from the mother until the completion of parturition. The ideal temperature for the young is 25–30°C (77–86°F), easily obtained with the aid of a heater.

2. Cutting the umbilical cord

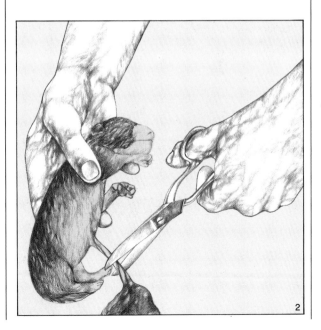

2

● Assessing the health of the young

● Make sure first of all that the young are still alive. If they are not obviously moving, try to observe their breathing and heartbeat (see pp. 98–99). If they are dead, remove them from the mother.
Weakly offspring must be kept warm, gently massaged and quickly submitted for veterinary attention.

● Checking growth

● Considering the fact that the majority of neo-natal deaths occur in the first 10–15 days of life, it is vital to keep a check on the growth and general health of the puppies and kittens during the first fortnight.
As well as ensuring that the vet is called to make a post-natal examination and subsequently at regular intervals, you should meanwhile weigh the young every two days on kitchen scales and record the results.
Normal, steady growth is the best sign of good health; the weight should have doubled within 7–10 days.
If an animal stops growing or loses weight, especially if you notice that it appears weak, call the vet at once.

LACTATION

Both cats and dogs produce milk for least 6–8 weeks after giving birth, until the young are weaned. The amount produced gradually increases in line with the growth of the young, until 4–5 weeks after the birth when it reduces.
The main problems at this stage can be:

● Eclampsia

● Eclampsia is a serious disorder which can occur in bitches from the end of pregnancy to the end of weaning (most commonly 3–6 weeks after giving birth) and less often in cats (about 2–4 weeks into lactation).
The early signs are a state of apprehension followed by involuntary muscular contractions that become increasingly stronger and often eventually result in long spasms and convulsions.
It is caused by the calcium losses in the milk which the body cannot replace sufficiently rapidly. This lowers the blood calcium level, and once it is below a certain level these signs will appear.
Call the vet at once, since the condition can prove fatal but is easily cured with the right treatment.

● Insufficient or no milk (agalactia)

This condition may be suspected if puppies or kittens are upset (restless, crying, cold) because suckling produces no milk. You should promptly call the vet so he can prescribe a replacement diet for the young and treat the mother if possible.

If milk is merely insufficient, this is harder to assess, but it must be considered if the young are only gaining weight slowly even if they seem lively and in good health.

INVOLUTION OF THE UTERUS

After parturition, the uterus gradually goes back to its former size.

In the first 3–4 weeks, a vaginal discharge may occur, which is at first dark reddish, liquid and copious, and then gradually reduces, disappearing after the third to fourth week.

The main uterine conditions occurring after birth that need prompt attention by a vet are bleeding, infection and prolapse.

● Uterine bleeding

Uterine bleeding mainly occurs in the first few days after birth, and can be due to lesions suffered during the expulsion of foetuses. Bleeding could also be caused by involution.

● Infection

If the placentas or dead foetuses are retained, or lesions are sustained during parturition, bacteria may become established in the uterus. This can produce severe infection marked by fever, depression and a vaginal discharge with dark blood and pus, often evil smelling. If not treated at once, this may be fatal.

● Prolapsed uterus

During or after giving birth, the uterus, having undergone severe contractions in the expulsion of the young and the placentas, may prolapse. This means it turns inside out and protrudes from the vulva, wholly or in part. It is visible as a dark red mass, often dripping blood and hanging from the opening.

Keep the mass clean and protected with a dampened, clean cloth while taking the animal to the vet. Follow the same instructions as those for abdominal organs protruding from stomach wounds as explained on page 105.

FIRST AID FOR SMALL MAMMALS AND BIRDS

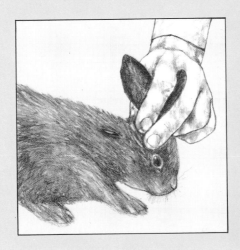

EMERGENCIES WITH SMALL MAMMALS

The most common small mammals kept as pets are rabbits, hamsters, guinea pigs, gerbils and mice.

Although cats and dogs hold a special place in our hearts and are the animals most commonly kept as pets, there are many small mammals that are becoming more and more popular with animal lovers, both young and old.

Less demanding than the traditional pet and having few special needs as regards environment and food, these smaller pets can be just as pleasing to those that dedicate a little time each day to their care. Rabbits, hamsters and guinea pigs make good pets if they are looked after well. They enjoy human company and appreciate being shown affection.

You need to pay attention to their health and deal with any illness in ways appropriate to their size and temperament.

Lastly, it should be remembered that small mammals generally have a fairly short life span: hamsters 2–3 years; mice 1–2 years; guinea pigs 5–6 years. When giving one to a child as a present, you should therefore bear in mind the inevitable upset that its loss will cause.

Emergencies with these animals are often the result of clumsy mistakes due to ignorance about the care of such pets. It is, therefore, best to find out about the particular needs of each species in order to appreciate their company fully.

Injuries

■ Injuries can be a common occurrence in the lives of dogs and cats but are far rarer in small mammals. This is because these smaller pets are generally confined to cages and therefore not able to move about freely. Also, they have a much more flexible bone structure ensuring less damage as a result of injury.

However, there are a few typical circumstances in which the animal's safety is put at risk, due usually to a lack of human awareness.

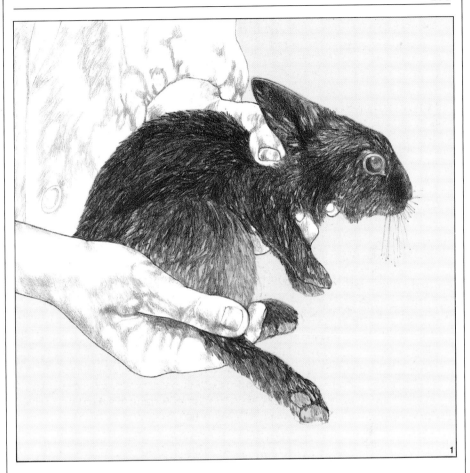

1. Examining the hind leg of a rabbit for a possible fracture

– Hamsters, guinea pigs and rabbits are often put up on tables just to be watched or played with. This may frighten the animal and lead to falls which can cause serious injury.

– The long claws of these animals can become entangled in the structure of a poorly constructed cage and cause injury.

– The use of exercise wheels or other metal toys in the cage is best avoided as they can injure the limbs and the tail.

Naturally, not all such accidents are predictable. If the worst happens, take action at once to catch the animal and restrain it.

■ Bone injuries

■ Losing the use of a limb because it is broken is serious for a small mammal so, if you suspect there is damage, you should gently palpate the bones to check for swellings and abnormal movement (fig. 1 on previous page).

Also, check for infected wounds under the coats which can be quite thick, as these can lead to problems if they are not treated.

Do not try to force an injured animal to take water or solid food. It may well not want it and, also, internal injury could become worse through ingestion of food.

■ Wounds

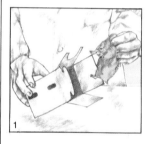

1. How to transport an injured small mammal
2. Skin injury
3. Disinfecting a skin injury

■ More common than bone injuries are the wounds, and in particular bites, which may occur when animals are housed together in small spaces (fig. 2 and 3).

A typical case is the hamster, normally a solitary animal, which will become very aggressive if housed with others.

An injured animal should be isolated at once. After doing so wait a few minutes to let the animal calm down and to avoid you receiving painful bites. Then examine the wounds, cutting back the haircoat at the edges for better access.

If there are deep and piercing injuries that might affect internal organs and structures (pleura, peritoneum etc.), it is best to confine the animal in a small container (see fig. 1) and take it to the vet at once.

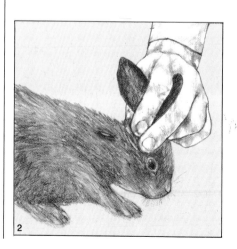

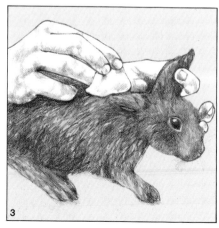

Physically caused emergencies

Often small mammals kept as pets are given insufficient attention and problems arise because of the poor conditions they are kept in.

■ **Heatstroke**

■ Heatstroke may develop in summer as a result of putting cages outside in the garden or on balconies in direct sunlight or leaving animals in cars during holiday trips. Many mammals, for example hamsters, live in the shade and must never be put into direct sunlight. The treatment for heatstroke is the same as for cats and dogs (see p. 136).

■ **Injuries from the cold**

■ Injuries due to cold are rare and almost exclusively affect mice and rats, which need a fairly high environmental temperature.
If a mouse cage is accidentally left outside on a cold evening, the mice may suffer from hypothermia. If this occurs, do not put them near powerful heat sources and avoid rubbing which will be useless and harmful; simply bring the animals inside and keep them at normal room temperature where they will recover in a few minutes.

Chemically caused emergencies

The use of various chemical products around the house, in ever-increasing quantities, means that extra care should be taken to avoid pets being poisoned.

■ **Poisoning**

■ Poisoning of caged animals is generally due to the careless use of insecticides in the form of sprays, powders and lotions, or the use of toxic household disinfectants and cleaning agents, or creosote on cages. The signs of poisoning can vary greatly. The animals can be lifeless or trembling, and may suffer from vomiting or diarrhea.
If you think the animal ingested the poison only a few minutes ago, try to make the animal vomit by giving it a few drops of saturated salt solution. If, on the other hand, the ingestion occurred some hours ago, only a vet can help, but you must tell him what substances may have been ingested or given to the animal in the last few hours.

Gastro-intestinal emergencies

Most gastro-intestinal emergencies are similar in all mammals but we will confine ourselves to those aspects relating to the smaller species in this section.

■ Foreign bodies

■ Rabbits and guinea pigs may suffer from foreign bodies becoming stuck between the roof of the mouth (front teeth) and upper incisors (see fig. 1). Usually, this is caused by vegetable matter which is too fibrous to be chewed but which the animals will nevertheless readily eat.

Signs include excessive salivation with constant attempts at swallowing and extreme nervousness in the animal. The material may have been dislodged by the repeated mouth movements, and have passed further down to obstruct the larynx or penetrate the surrounding tissue. This can have grave consequences and prompt examination of the guinea pig's or rabbit's mouth under a good source of light will be required.

Similarly, if there is wire around the teeth or, worse still, around the tongue which as a result may be swollen and painful, check the mouth carefully. If you find the animal is too restless to allow intervention, do not try force but take it to the vet who may be able to deal with the problem after giving an anaesthetic.

1. Extraction of a foreign body from the mouth

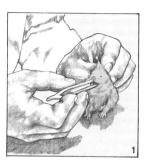

■ Damage to the teeth

■ With guinea pigs there can be damage to the teeth, above all to the incisors (long front teeth) which grow too long through an incorrect diet and then break at the base with some degree of bleeding. This limits the animal's eating, and its physical decline is then swift. It helps to shorten the remaining incisors with clippers so that food can be picked up again with the teeth.

■ Abdominal gas

■ The presence of gas in the abdomen causes severe distention. The signs are depression and abdominal pain.

All forms must be assessed promptly by checking the faeces and urine in the cage for any abnormality. Look to see whether there is any bleeding from the anus or in the urine.

If you cannot make an accurate judgement, it is a

good idea to use paper instead of normal bedding; this will make it easier to examine what the animal is passing.

■ **Constipation**

■ Constipation is often due to masses of vegetable material collecting in the anal canal. These are easily removed with plastic tweezers.

■ **Prolapsed rectum**

■ Hamsters, mice and rats may suffer from a prolapsed rectum. It makes the animal very agitated and lack appetite. It will constantly turn to lick or bite the prolapsed part which looks like a red bit of string protruding from the anus.

Any attempt at pushing this back is useless. You should moisten the part with tepid water and put the pet into a small cage with cloth or paper on the floor.

You will then need to seek the help of a vet at once.

Breathing emergencies

Only occasionally are there sudden and dramatic breathing emergencies with small mammals.

■ **Asthma**

■ Hamsters and gerbils sometimes show signs of asthma, especially young ones or those expending too much energy or in stressful situations. Sneezing and breathing difficulties will disappear in a few hours if the animal is not handled but left in its cage in peace.

■ **Pneumonia**

■ Respiratory tract infections are possible in all small mammals. They may progress to pneumonia with heaving, open-mouthed breathing. The animal is too distressed to be able to feed and veterinary attention is imperative. Keep the animal warm in the meantime.

Neurological emergencies

Other than the emergencies common to all mammals, there are some conditions peculiar to certain small mammals.

■ **Convulsive fits**

■ Young mice and gerbils may suffer convulsive

fits, with limbs trembling and rigid. Such fits tend to vanish as the animal grows older and learns to trust humans.

■ **Cage paralysis**

■ So-called "cage paralysis" is due to vitamin D deficiency and a lack of exercise; the animal moves slowly and finds it hard to hold up its head. A multivitamin supplement and a bigger cage will solve the trouble.

■ **Lethargy**

■ Hamsters normally go into hibernation and even in captivity may show lethargy and torpor, seeming almost lifeless. Gentle massage with a woollen cloth will revive the animal.

Obstetrical emergencies

As with all animals, emergencies can arise during pregnancy and birth in small mammals.

■ **Toxaemia**

■ In rabbits and guinea pigs, toxaemia may occur in the final stages of pregnancy; the animal seems listless, hardly reacting to stimuli and sometimes showing a slight vaginal discharge. In a case of toxaemia do not delay as the animal may die within a few hours unless a Caesarian operation is performed.

■ **Uterine inertia**

■ Rabbits and guinea pigs may delay giving birth, retaining the foetuses.
Observe the animal carefully before and after giving birth to check that it is in good shape, taking an interest in feeding its young, and actively cleaning itself.

Below is a list of the gestation periods of the small mammals in days.

Rabbit	30
Guinea pig	65 – 71
Mouse	20
Rat	21
Hamster	16
Squirrel	37
Chinchilla	105 –115
Gerbil	24 – 26

EMERGENCIES WITH BIRDS

T *the most common cage birds are budgerigars, canaries, cockatoos, small African and Australian finches, talking parrots and Indian Minah birds.*

Injuries

Injuries are generally caused by the cage accidentally falling over or by sudden frights, attacks by cats, and in the case of pigeons, collisions with cars. The immediate consequences can be broken wings or feet.

In the case of fractures, you should first of all check whether the overlying skin is broken and the fracture is exposed or not. If part of a bone is exposed, take the animal to a vet at once. If not, you can try to reduce the fracture by immobilizing the bird.

■ **Broken foot**

■ For a foot fracture, you can use the quill of a big feather from a pigeon or hen cut lengthwise and as long as the leg. Once it is in position fix it to the leg with adhesive plaster (fig. 1). This is an effective splint which should be left in place for up to 20 days.

1. Treatment of fractured limb:
a) preparation of a quill
b) application

1. Immobilization of a
fractured wing: a) applying
the plaster; b) tying the wings

■ Broken wing

■ Entangled legs

During this time the bird should be kept in a small
cage without a perch and with brown paper (not
sand paper) on the floor.

■ For a broken wing you can use a plaster of soap
mixed with white of egg. This is applied under the
wing between it and the body. When it is well fixed,
tie the two wing ends together (fig. 1). Then keep
the animal in the same way as with a broken foot.

■ In towns and cities pigeons' legs sometimes get
entangled in wire or string, preventing their movement and threatening to cut off their claws.
In such cases cut the string with fine scissors, such

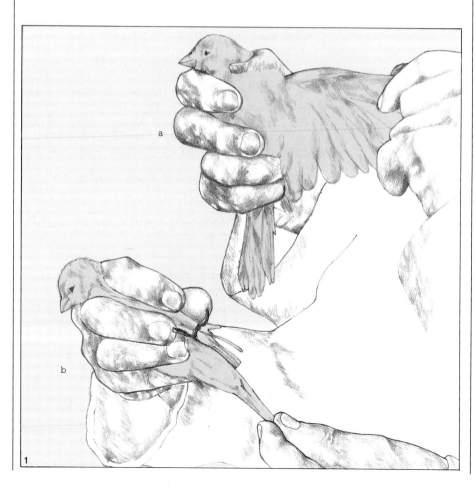

as small sewing scissors, taking care not to damage the vital part of the foot. The foot is usually swollen because of the constricting string so that the part to be cut can be deeply hidden in the flesh. Slowly introduce the scissors and cut the string. Sometimes blood appears, but this is usually not a risk to the bird. You should simply disinfect the area with an ordinary antiseptic agent, and the wound will quickly heal. During this time, keep the bird in a clean place to avoid infection of the freshly exposed wound.

Physically caused emergencies

■ **Heatstroke**

■ The most common occurrence of heatstroke is when a cage is exposed directly to the sun. Sunlight as such is not harmful to birds, but they should always be able to seek shelter from it. When you put a cage outside make sure that it is half covered with a piece of cloth. The bird can then choose either to be in the sun or shade.

With heatstroke, a bird will be distressed and lie prostrate on the bottom of its cage. It will move sluggishly as if dazed. The body temperature will be very high.

Gently pick up the bird, dip its head in cold water several times and see how it reacts; normally it will begin to move again after a short while. At this stage, return it to its cage in a cool spot that is dark and quiet. Usually, in a few hours the bird will recover.

■ **Hypothermia**

■ Another emergency that may occur with birds in cages is hypothermia. It can be caused by a sudden storm. If the cage has been left in the open, the bird may be drenched causing a sudden fall in body temperature.

When you find it, its appearance may be alarming. To remedy the situation, wrap the bird in blotting paper or absorbent kitchen towel to dry the feathers as best as you can. A hair drier may be used if held sufficiently far away. Such birds will re-open their eyes and gradually move as their feathers become dry and their bodies warm. Keep them wrapped for a while longer in a piece of woollen cloth that has been slightly warmed with an iron and then return them to their cage in a sheltered spot. This usually achieves recovery without after effects.

Abdominal emergencies

Abdominal emergencies are often caused by enteritis or hepatitis. An affected bird shows ruffled feathers, listless behaviour and lack of appetite, as well as dirty feathers in the anal region. The disease is normally caused by a defective diet or by contaminated bird seed, or insufficiently washed and dried greenstuff.

■ **Hepatitis**

■ To assess what organ is affected, take the bird in hand and gently blow on its abdominal feathers to examine the skin. If you find a dark spot on the right side, it is an indication of a swollen liver. This requires attention from the vet who will prescribe drugs and a proper diet.

■ **Enteritis**

■ If the abdomen is swollen and hurts when palpated, it suggests a case of enteritis. This may be curable by adding lemon juice to the drinking water and barring fruit and greens from the diet for at least 10 days. If the general state of the bird is more serious, the vet will prescribe a course of drugs.

Breathing emergencies

Respiratory illnesses are not always easy to diagnose (asthma, catarrh, chronic breathing sickness etc.). If a bird appears to be suffering from laboured breathing, you will need to consult a vet for the correct treatment.

Obstetrical emergencies

■ **Laying of eggs**

■ When the nest is finished, the female usually lays one egg a day for 3–6 days. Check in the morning whether an egg has been laid, by gently coaxing the female from the nest. A canary will readily respond to this and then quietly return to the nest. If instead, the bird is anxious and depressed, fails to leave the nest and stays put with eyes closed, the reason may well be that the egg has not yet been laid and is still in the cloaca.

To check whether this is so, hold the bird gently as shown in figure 1 and with a finger palpate the abdomen. If there is an egg, you will easily be able to feel it.

■ **Difficulty in laying**

■ To induce the laying of the egg, boil a saucepan of water. Take the bird and expose it to the vapour as shown in figure 2. After 10 minutes, stop the treatment, wrap the bird in a cloth and leave it alone. After ½–1 hour check to see if the egg has been laid. If it has not, take the bird to a vet at once.

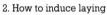

1. How to see if there is an unlaid egg
2. How to induce laying

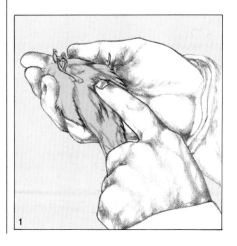

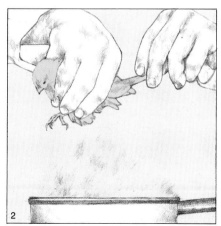

APPENDIX

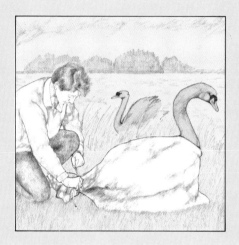

REPRODUCTION

This section deals with reproduction in cats and dogs and how to recognize some of the problems that may arise.

The first-aid measures to be applied in cases of labour and post-partum difficulties are described in the chapter on obstetrical emergencies on page 185.

Sexual cycle in dogs

■ **Puberty**

■ A bitch reaches sexual maturity, with the first oestrus, at 6–12 months. This usually occurs 2 months before reaching full size; small dogs, therefore, become mature and enter puberty earlier than large ones.

■ **Oestrous cycles**

■ From puberty bitches are "on heat" at regular intervals. In most cases there are two oestrous cycles a year with intervals of approximately 6 months. However, in some breeds there is only one, such as in Basenjis.

It is useful to note the dates of the cycle to have an idea of the regularity and know roughly when to expect the next heat. However, there can be considerable variation in the length of the interval between successive heats and supposed "irregularity" is by no means abnormal. However, repeated excessively early or late heats should be mentioned to the vet.

In bitches, the cycle does not stop at a later stage in life (as is the case in humans), but with age it may become less frequent or less obvious.

■ **Phases of the oestrous cycle**

■ The oestrous cycle in bitches is made up of four phases: pro-oestrus; oestrus; dioestrus and metoestrus; anoestrus.

Pro-oestrus

This phase is marked by a blood-stained discharge from the vulva. The vulva itself will appear enlarged. Some days before the discharge is apparent, there may be some change in behaviour and the bitch will seem quieter than usual. During the pro-oestrus, however, she may become distinctly nervous.

	In this phase, bitches will not mate and can be aggressive to males. Males are attracted by the smell of the vaginal secretion and there is increasing interest between the two sexes. The phase ends as discharge gradually stops and males are then accepted. It usually lasts from 3–16 days, but on average 9 days.
Oestrus	The bitch is ready to mate, showing this in the presence of a male by drawing the tail to one side and exposing the vulva. The vulva remains enlarged but is softer to allow penetration. The vaginal discharge changes in colour from blood-stained to clear. Also during this phase, the bitch may try to escape from its home in order to mate. The combination of pro-oestrus and oestrus, commonly referred to as the "heat," lasts about 3 weeks.
Diostrus and metoestrus	This phase begins after the bitch stops accepting males and the vulva starts to return to its normal dimensions. Although a few days after this phase the bitch may seem to be back to "normal," it takes much longer until progesterone production finally stops, from 30–90 days.
Anoestrus	This is the resting phase and the oestrus cycle is quiescent until the next one begins. The length of anoestrus will be related to the frequency of the heat periods the bitch has in the year.
■ **Abnormal cases**	■ Certain abnormal situations related to the course of the oestrus cycle may arise and these need the attention of the vet.
Abnormal length of phases	A phase which is excessively longer or shorter than the lengths indicated may indicate that the ovaries are undergoing changes.
False pregnancy	This term refers to the late phase (dioestrus and metoestrus) when signs similar to pregnancy and/or giving birth may appear. During this phase of the oestrus cycle hormonal balance is similar to that in actual pregnancy. In some bitches, overt signs of a false pregnancy may appear some days after oestrus, usually after 30–90 days, and may be apparent for another 2–3 weeks.

As happens at the end of a true pregnancy the teats are enlarged and secrete first a clear fluid and then milk, which readily flows on compressing them.

Behaviour can be abnormal, such as seeking a suitable spot for giving birth, maternal behaviour towards objects such as toys and cushions, increased appetite and sometimes genuine pains.

It is advisable to call the vet to exclude the possibility of a true pregnancy and so that you can be given advice on how to deal with the condition.

Pyometra

Pyometra is a serious condition, found mainly in middle-aged and older bitches and during metoestrus, from 2 weeks after the end of heat.

It is caused by the uterus which, while ready to receive and nurture the developing young animals, becomes infected by bacteria.

Signs are various degrees of depression, reduction or absence of appetite, increased thirst and urine production and sometimes vomiting. Often there is a discharge from the vulva (so-called "open" cases), containing mucus, pus and at times blood, appearing from creamy-yellow to blood-tinged.

If any of these signs are noticed, especially in the phase indicated, you should seek help from the vet who will decide on the correct therapy, medical or surgical.

Mating

The male is attracted to the female mainly by the smell of certain substances present in the vaginal secretion, and possibly in the anal glands, of a bitch on heat.

Mating is preceded by a brief "courtship" stage in which the male smells and licks the female's vulva.

A female, if receptive, will draw the tail sideways; if not she may rebel, become aggressive and seek to escape.

Mating in dogs is made up of two stages. In the initial phase, the male mounts the bitch and introduces the partially erect penis into the vagina by means of a series of pelvic thrusts as seen in figure 1a; erection quickly becomes complete causing dilatation of the bulb. This is a thicker part of the penis some distance from the tip which is held by contraction of the vaginal muscles in an arrangement which prevents the penis from slipping out. After thrusting, the male dismounts but does not disconnect. He will turn round and lift one hind leg over the bitch until he reaches the position shown in figure 1b; this "copulatory tie" is maintained for 20–25 minutes until the erection subsides.

Emission of sperm occurs shortly after insertion, at the end of thrusting.

■ Undesirable matings

■ While every attempt should be made to avoid a bitch roaming free when she is on heat, unfortunately it can sometimes happen that a bitch is

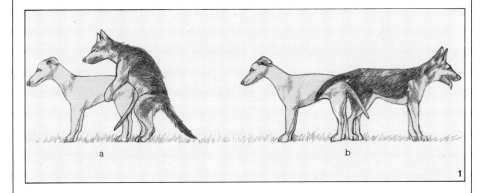

1. Mating in dogs:
a) first stage
b) second stage

mounted against the owner's wishes.

If the owner sees this happening, an attempt may be made to separate the dogs, but this can only be done before penetration has taken place. After that it would be very difficult because of the dilatation of the bulb. In fact it would be very painful for the dogs and could cause permanent injury. It would also not remedy the situation as the most crucial emission of sperm occurs very early on.

If you intervene too late, it is therefore best to let the dogs carry on and call the vet so that a drug to prevent conception may be given. It should be remembered that these drugs are only effective if given in the first 2–3 days after mating.

To prevent such matings, it helps to know roughly when the heat should start and to look for the first blood-stained discharge. Once the heat has begun, keep the bitch away from other dogs and on a lead when she absolutely must be taken out. Do not leave her to roam freely even if she seems to reject males as some bitches will accept mating before the blood-stained discharge disappears.

Sexual cycles in cats

■ **Puberty**

■ Cats begin to be on heat at 6–12 months of age, but sometimes earlier or later. Sexual maturity will depend on the speed of growth, (although this is fairly similar in all cats), breed (long-coated breeds are often later) and the time of year they were born, since coming into heat must coincide with the reproductive season for cats.

The cycles continue until an advanced age, when they may become irregular or stop.

■ **Oestrous cycle**

■ Cats show signs of being on heat several times a year during their breeding season. The length of the season depends mainly on the number of hours of daylight. In Europe it varies between January and October; in northern Europe and Britain it begins in January and ends in September.

■ **Phases of the cycle**

■ The same four phases make up the oestrous in cats as in dogs.

Pro-oestrus

This lasts for 1–3 days only, without any special signs such as discharge or a swollen vulva. Sometimes there is a slight change in behaviour and the cat is perhaps more affectionate and sometimes more restless.

Oestrus

The cat shows a clear change in behaviour during this phase; the characteristic "calling" is a feature, as is taking up a mating position with tail drawn to the side, forelimbs lowered and hind quarters raised up, and at times rubbing and rolling on the back; often there is loss of appetite.

This phase lasts from a few days to two weeks, depending on whether mating does or does not occur. Ova (eggs) to be fertilized are not released spontaneously as in humans and dogs, but as a result of the stimulus of intercourse.

Signs of heat will stop some two days after mating,

but if this does not take place, they will continue until the end of the oestrus phase.
Unmated cats will soon return to pro-oestrus.

Dioestrus and metoestrus

If there has been ovulation but no successful fertilization, this phase may last 1–2 months and involve a false pregnancy, as occurs with dogs.

Anoestrus

This is the resting phase during the period of diminished daylight when the ovaries are inactive. The number of yearly oestrous cycles in a cat depends on the length of the breeding season and on the length of individual cycles. With fertilization and subsequent pregnancy, the cycles are interrupted until the kittens are weaned.
Sometimes the next heat may return even earlier, even one week after giving birth, especially if the kittens have been removed. Heat can also occasionally appear in the early stages of pregnancy, around about the third week; if mating takes place and fertilization occurs, the cat will have developing young of different ages in the uterus.

■ Abnormal conditions

■ The main disturbances of the cycle which will need the help of a vet are:

Nymphomania

With this condition a cat shows signs of severe and continuous heat, which may be due to ovarian cysts. It can also happen that cats remain on heat continuously (for example, if exposed to sufficient artificial light) and show exaggerated behaviour without abnormal ovaries.

False pregnancy

A cat, after a sterile mating may show signs of a false pregnancy, with behaviour typical of late pregnancy and early post-partum stages. In comparison to dogs, in the cats the teats are less often enlarged and milk is more rarely secreted.
This condition is not regarded as a disease and no treatment is needed.

Pyometra

Pyometra is caused by infection, mainly in the late phase (dioestrus), especially after an infertile coupling. In this phase the uterus undergoes certain changes that make it particularly susceptible to infection.
The main symptoms are a loss of appetite and

interest, increased thirst and urination and sometimes a vaginal discharge.
Cats showing one or more of these symptoms, especially in the phase following heat, should be seen
immediately by the vet.

Mating

The male is attracted to the female by two features:
by smell, through the production of certain substances, known as pheromones, eliminated in the
urine; or by behaviour patterns such as calling,
treading movements and positions indicating an
excited state.
When a male is present, the female miaows more
intensely, rubs her head on any nearby object,
turns nervously and takes up a mating stance with
raised hips and tail drawn sideways.

The male mounts the female, as illustrated in
figure 1. Mating is swift and the male leaves at once
to escape the often violent reactions of the female.
After the first mating several more matings tend to
follow, often with different partners if the animals
are free to roam. This may lead to fertilization by
two or more tomcats.

Pregnancy in cats and dogs

■ **Duration**

■ In dogs pregnancy lasts 63 days on average and
the majority of births take place after 60–66 days.
Pregnancies lasting between 55–71 days are considered normal.
In cats the average length of pregnancy is 64–65
days, and those lasting between 58–71 days are
considered normal.
The gestation (pregnancy) table on page 220 allows
you to work out the most likely date of birth. Each
date is shown alongside that of the first mating. In
leap years subtract 1 day for a birth expected from
1 March to 2 May.

■ **Bodily changes**

■ Both in cats and dogs, bodily changes become
evident halfway through pregnancy. In the second
half of pregnancy, about 5–6 weeks, the abdomen

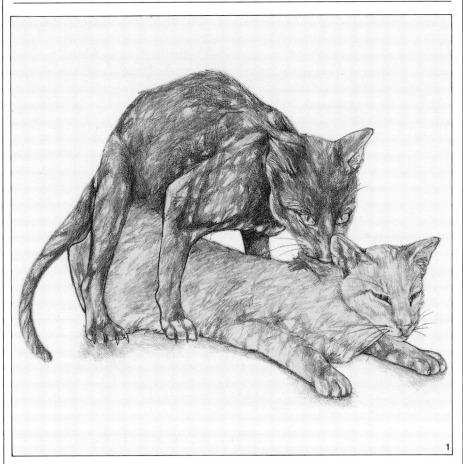

1. Mating in cats

gradually swells and the teats become bigger, though often only in the last week in cats.

■ Abortions

■ Both in cats and dogs, abortions may occur spontaneously, often for reasons hard to establish.

The signs of an abortion are vaginal leakage, often with blood and expulsion of foetuses and fragments of foetal membrane in advanced cases.

If dead foetuses are not expelled it will result in their decomposition and the development of toxaemia. The animal will be very depressed, with increases in thirst and urination, fever and often a foul dark vaginal discharge. If this is the case, veterinary attention is essential.

Giving birth

■ Early signs

■ It is important to be able to recognize early signs in order to help effectively at the moment of giving birth.

Dogs

One or two days beforehand, some obvious changes in behaviour may occur. The bitch often seeks a place in which to give birth, perhaps digging in her basket with her paws. She displays anxiety, trembling and possibly seeking her owner's affection. Sometimes appetite will drop and thirst increase. The teats may begin to secrete milk.

The most common sign of imminent parturition in bitches is a drop in temperature from 38.5°C to about 37.5°C (101.5 to 99.5°F), from 15–20 hours beforehand. Therefore, it is a good idea to check the rectal temperature after 55 days of pregnancy twice a day (see p. 54).

Cats

In a cat the early signs are far less obvious. The fall in body temperature is not so marked or consistent. In the last week, the animal becomes quieter and may begin to occupy the most suitable spot for the birth of its young. At the same time the teats become more prominent. In the final days, appetite may drop. Clear changes in behaviour only occur just before the moment of giving birth. Some cats become aggressive towards people they do not know and others wish to be close to their owner. Generally, they display signs of uneasiness, sometimes revealed by miaowing.

■ Stages of labour

■ Giving birth includes two main stages followed by a third stage when the foetal membranes are expelled.

First stage

The first stage can last some hours and prepares for the expulsion of the young with the dilation of the neck of the uterus.
The animal may be particularly calm or somewhat excited, refuse food and often inspect its own flanks. At the end of this phase the first obvious contractions of the uterus begin.

Second stage

Each of the young is expelled following strong contractions. First the allantoic fluid escapes, after rupture of the first membrane. Next, the amniotic sac (water bag) will appear at the vulva (see illustration on page 218). If it does not break, the mother will tear it and clear fluid is released. Finally, the young animal appears at the exit of the birth canal. If forelegs and head or hind legs and tail appear first, the presentation is normal. Once the puppy or kitten appears, straining a few more times will normally bring it out completely (see illustration on page 219).

Third stage

The foetal membranes are expelled, either after each young animal is born, or collectively after the birth of a few, or all together right at the end.

The first stage is common to all species, the others are repeated several times in multiparous species (those normally producing more than one offspring).
In dogs the normal interval between births varies from a few minutes to an hour, being shorter earlier and longer later. In some litters it may be up to more than 2 hours. A normal parturition should not exceed 12 hours and usually it is completed in 2–6 hours.
In cats the intervals are of the same length as dogs, but can be more irregular.
Often 2 or 3 kittens are expelled in quick succession, with a long pause of 2 hours or more afterwards.
Sometimes there is a physiological block, lasting up to a day (even 2 days in a cat), in which the bitch or cat rests, behaving as if parturition were finished, looking after the young and cleaning herself; afterwards renewed straining begins and the rest of the litter is born.

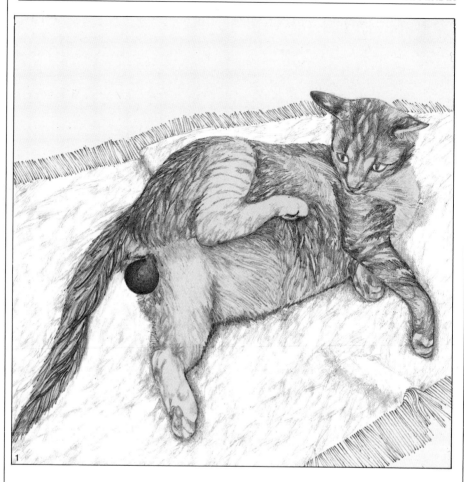

Second stage of a cat giving
birth: the amniotic sac at the
vulva

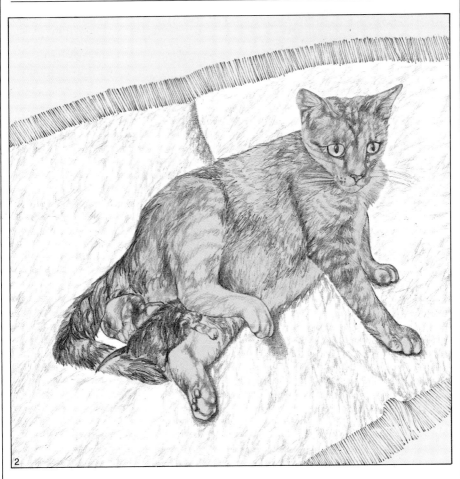

2

Second stage of a cat giving
birth: kitten appearing at the
exit of the birth canal

Table of pregnancies
calculated on an average of
63 days

JAN		FEB		MAR		APR		MAY		JUNE	
1	5 MAR	1	5 APR	1	3 MAY	1	3 JUN	1	3 JUL	1	3 AUG
2	6 MAR	2	6 APR	2	4 MAY	2	4 JUN	2	4 JUL	2	4 AUG
3	7 MAR	3	7 APR	3	5 MAY	3	5 JUN	3	5 JUL	3	5 AUG
4	8 MAR	4	8 APR	4	6 MAY	4	6 JUN	4	6 JUL	4	6 AUG
5	9 MAR	5	9 APR	5	7 MAY	5	7 JUN	5	7 JUL	5	7 AUG
6	10 MAR	6	10 APR	6	8 MAY	6	8 JUN	6	8 JUL	6	8 AUG
7	11 MAR	7	11 APR	7	9 MAY	7	9 JUN	7	9 JUL	7	9 AUG
8	12 MAR	8	12 APR	8	10 MAY	8	10 JUN	8	10 JUL	8	10 AUG
9	13 MAR	9	13 APR	9	11 MAY	9	11 JUN	9	11 JUL	9	11 AUG
10	14 MAR	10	14 APR	10	12 MAY	10	12 JUN	10	12 JUL	10	12 AUG
11	15 MAR	11	15 APR	11	13 MAY	11	13 JUN	11	13 JUL	11	13 AUG
12	16 MAR	12	16 APR	12	14 MAY	12	14 JUN	12	14 JUL	12	14 AUG
13	17 MAR	13	17 APR	13	15 MAY	13	15 JUN	13	15 JUL	13	15 AUG
14	18 MAR	14	18 APR	14	16 MAY	14	16 JUN	14	16 JUL	14	16 AUG
15	19 MAR	15	19 APR	15	17 MAY	15	17 JUN	15	17 JUL	15	17 AUG
16	20 MAR	16	20 APR	16	18 MAY	16	18 JUN	16	18 JUL	16	18 AUG
17	21 MAR	17	21 APR	17	19 MAY	17	19 JUN	17	19 JUL	17	19 AUG
18	22 MAR	18	22 APR	18	20 MAY	18	20 JUN	18	20 JUL	18	20 AUG
19	23 MAR	19	23 APR	19	21 MAY	19	21 JUN	19	21 JUL	19	21 AUG
20	24 MAR	20	24 APR	20	22 MAY	20	22 JUN	20	22 JUL	20	22 AUG
21	25 MAR	21	25 APR	21	23 MAY	21	23 JUN	21	23 JUL	21	23 AUG
22	26 MAR	22	26 APR	22	24 MAY	22	24 JUN	22	24 JUL	22	24 AUG
23	27 MAR	23	27 APR	23	25 MAY	23	25 JUN	23	25 JUL	23	25 AUG
24	28 MAR	24	28 APR	24	26 MAY	24	26 JUN	24	26 JUL	24	26 AUG
25	29 MAR	25	29 APR	25	27 MAY	25	27 JUN	25	27 JUL	25	27 AUG
26	30 MAR	26	30 APR	26	28 MAY	26	28 JUN	26	28 JUL	26	28 AUG
27	31 MAR	27	1 MAY	27	29 MAY	27	29 JUN	27	29 JUL	27	29 AUG
28	1 APR	28	2 MAY	28	30 MAY	28	30 JUN	28	30 JUL	28	30 AUG
29	2 APR	29	3 MAY	29	31 MAY	29	1 JUL	29	31 JUL	29	31 AUG
30	3 APR			30	1 JUN	30	2 JUL	30	1 AUG	30	1 SEP
31	4 APR			31	2 JUN			31	2 AUG		

	JUL		AUG		SEP		OCT		NOV		DEC
1	2 SEP	1	3 OCT	1	3 NOV	1	3 DEC	1	3 JAN	1	2 FEB
2	3 SEP	2	4 OCT	2	4 NOV	2	4 DEC	2	4 JAN	2	3 FEB
3	4 SEP	3	5 OCT	3	5 NOV	3	5 DEC	3	5 JAN	3	4 FEB
4	5 SEP	4	6 OCT	4	6 NOV	4	6 DEC	4	6 JAN	4	5 FEB
5	6 SEP	5	7 OCT	5	7 NOV	5	7 DEC	5	7 JAN	5	6 FEB
6	7 SEP	6	8 OCT	6	8 NOV	6	8 DEC	6	8 JAN	6	7 FEB
7	8 SEP	7	9 OCT	7	9 NOV	7	9 DEC	7	9 JAN	7	8 FEB
8	9 SEP	8	10 OCT	8	10 NOV	8	10 DEC	8	10 JAN	8	9 FEB
9	10 SEP	9	11 OCT	9	11 NOV	9	11 DEC	9	11 JAN	9	10 FEB
10	11 SEP	10	12 OCT	10	12 NOV	10	12 DEC	10	12 JAN	10	11 FEB
11	12 SEP	11	13 OCT	11	13 NOV	11	13 DEC	11	13 JAN	11	12 FEB
12	13 SEP	12	14 OCT	12	14 NOV	12	14 DEC	12	14 JAN	12	13 FEB
13	14 SEP	13	15 OCT	13	15 NOV	13	15 DEC	13	15 JAN	13	14 FEB
14	15 SEP	14	16 OCT	14	16 NOV	14	16 DEC	14	16 JAN	14	15 FEB
15	16 SEP	15	17 OCT	15	17 NOV	15	17 DEC	15	17 JAN	15	16 FEB
16	17 SEP	16	18 OCT	16	18 NOV	16	18 DEC	16	18 JAN	16	17 FEB
17	18 SEP	17	19 OCT	17	19 NOV	17	19 DEC	17	19 JAN	17	18 FEB
18	19 SEP	18	20 OCT	18	20 NOV	18	20 DEC	18	20 JAN	18	19 FEB
19	20 SEP	19	21 OCT	19	21 NOV	19	21 DEC	19	21 JAN	19	20 FEB
20	21 SEP	20	22 OCT	20	22 NOV	20	22 DEC	20	22 JAN	20	21 FEB
21	22 SEP	21	23 OCT	21	23 NOV	21	23 DEC	21	23 JAN	21	22 FEB
22	23 SEP	22	24 OCT	22	24 NOV	22	24 DEC	22	24 JAN	22	23 FEB
23	24 SEP	23	25 OCT	23	25 NOV	23	25 DEC	23	25 JAN	23	24 FEB
24	25 SEP	24	26 OCT	24	26 NOV	24	26 DEC	24	26 JAN	24	25 FEB
25	26 SEP	25	27 OCT	25	27 NOV	25	27 DEC	25	27 JAN	25	26 FEB
26	27 SEP	26	28 OCT	26	28 NOV	26	28 DEC	26	28 JAN	26	27 FEB
27	28 SEP	27	29 OCT	27	29 NOV	27	29 DEC	27	29 JAN	27	28 FEB
28	29 SEP	28	30 OCT	28	30 NOV	28	30 DEC	28	30 JAN	28	1 MAR
29	30 SEP	29	31 OCT	29	1 DEC	29	31 DEC	29	31 JAN	29	2 MAR
30	1 OCT	30	1 NOV	30	2 DEC	30	1 JAN	30	1 FEB	30	3 MAR
31	2 OCT	31	2 NOV			31	2 JAN			31	4 MAR

RECOVERY
OF STRAYS

S ometimes, around
the town or in the
country, you might
come across a stray
animal: a wild cat, a lost
dog or a bird in distress.
This section offers some
advice on how to go
about helping them.

Cats and dogs

Finding a stray cat or dog (as indeed taking in or being given one) presents a series of practical problems. You should, above all, try to understand the immediate help the animal may need. This will depend on the physical characteristics and overall fitness of the animal in question. You can begin to have an idea of what treatment may be needed by answering three important questions.
– roughly how old is it?
– what sex is it?
– what is its state of health?

ASSESSING AGE

■ **Puppies and kittens**

■ The rate of growth during the first month is roughly similar in kittens and puppies.

First weeks

From birth up to 1–2 weeks old, puppies and kittens have eyes and ears shut, and no teeth (fig. 3). For the first few days remnants of the umbilical cord may be present.
After about 10 days, the eyes and ears open and the teeth appear after the third week. You will be able to reckon, therefore, that a puppy with a complete set of front teeth is at least one month old (fig. 1).

1

After 1 month

After 1 month the young become more active and their movements more co-ordinated. From 1 month up to 3½ months, at which point the milk teeth start to be replaced, age is harder to judge for the inexperienced. Between 2 and 3 months, dogs show a certain amount of wear on the incisors, the points becoming flattened (fig. 2). After 2 months, eye colour stabilizes.

2

After 3 months

After 3 months the milk teeth begin to be replaced, the first to be lost being the incisors beginning with

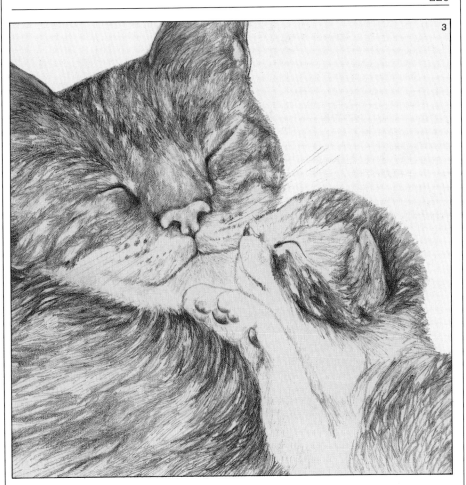

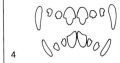

After 6–7 months

the innermost (fig. 4). At around 4–5 months old, all the incisors have been replaced, and between 5 and 6 months so have the canines.

After 6–7 months all the permanent teeth are in place (fig. 5). The animal gradually reaches adult size. In the male the external genitals grow to reach their final size between the ages of 9 and 12 months old.

■ Accurately gauging the age of an adult dog is difficult, and even more so of an adult cat. However, a rough estimate as to whether you are dealing with a

young animal, an adult animal or an old animal is possible.
To do this, you should examine the teeth, eyes and greying of the coat.

■ Teeth

■ The most important feature to examine is the teeth to see how healthy they are and if there is any decay.

Tartar deposits

Tartar deposits are found both in cats and dogs from about one year onwards. It is a slow process involving an accumulation of plaque at the base of the teeth, especially the canines, premolars and molars.
There is naturally a great deal of variation in the rate at which these tartar deposits develop. It will depend on the type of diet (wet or dry food), on the species in question and on inherited characteristics. However, as a general guideline, you can presume than an animal with obvious tartar will be older than 2–3 years old (fig. 1).
In animals later in life, generally those older than 10 years, the deposit may be brown and foul smelling and cover the teeth completely (fig. 2). In some cases affected teeth may even be loose and painful. However, you should bear in mind that an animal's teeth may have been cleaned regularly by a vet; in this case, a cat or dog may maintain a healthy-looking set of teeth well into old age and you will not be able to judge the age accurately from this feature.

1. Initial tartar deposits
2. Thick tartar deposits in an old dog

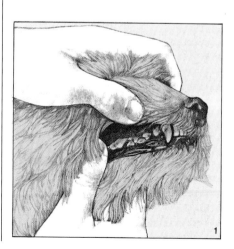
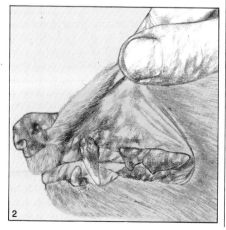

3. Loss of incisors

Tooth decay:
4. around 2 years
5. between 2 and 3 years
6. around 4 to 5 years

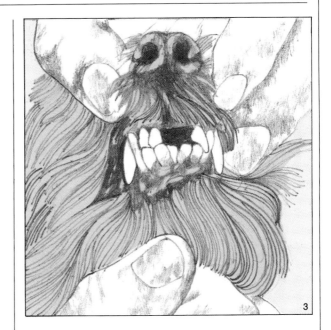

3

Wear of teeth

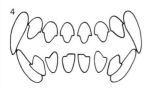

4

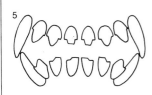

5

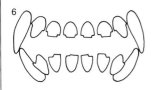

6

Loss of teeth

In the same way as with tartar deposits, the wear of teeth in dogs not only varies according to diet and behaviour (eating dry food or bones, gnawing stones and other hard objects), but also depends on the correct occlusion and apposition of the teeth.

In dogs, while bearing in mind the possibility of large individual variation, wear of teeth is judged by the notching and later the flattening of the most prominent point of the innermost two incisors (the upper ones normally have three cusps, the lower, two or three).

– After 1½ years, the two innermost upper canines begin to be worn and at 2 years old become flattened (fig. 4).

– The same changes can be seen to occur to the lower canines at 2–3 years old and to the upper ones at 4–5 (fig. 6).

In cats, the wear of teeth varies too much to be any indication of age.

The loss of teeth normally happens only in old age, that is after 11–12 years. Usually it is the incisors that are lost first (fig. 3).

■ Eyes

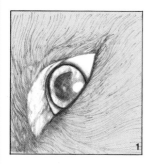

■ Greying

Aging in a dog:
1. lens becoming opaque
2. greying of coat

■ In a dog after 7 years, the eye may develop a small, clear blue–white rim round the iris which is most obvious at the top. When it first appears, it is thin but it thickens in time and becomes quite conspicuous after 10 years.

Again in adult dogs, you will be able to observe that the lens always becomes more opaque after the seventh or eighth year. This gives the pupillar opening an opalescent appearance (fig. 1). This development, known as "senile hardening of the lens" or "senile cataract" is normal and should present no cause for worry.

Of course, to rule out the possibility of cataract from other causes will require an examination by the vet.

■ You will only be able to observe greying in dogs with coloured coats. The first white hair usually appears on the chin and around the lips after about 6 years. It will then gradually spread upward to the cheeks and around the nose at 7–8 years, to the eyes at 8–9 years and the rest of the body after 10–11 years (fig. 2).

In cats this change is less evident.

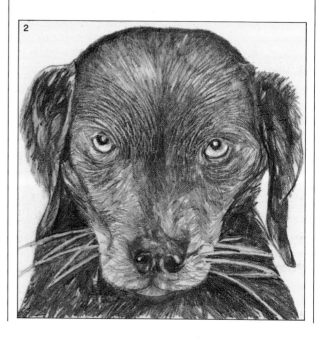

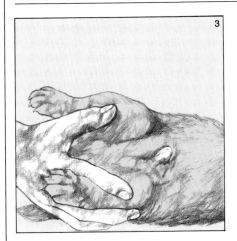

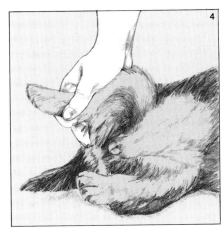

Puppies:
3. male
4. female

JUDGING SEX

In adult animals it is easy to recognize the sex since the external genital organs are well developed and instantly distinguishable.
On the other hand, in puppies and kittens, particularly those under one month old, it is more difficult.

To judge the sex in these cases, you should follow these simple instructions.

■ **Dog**

■ Lay the puppy on its back, spread its back legs and examine the abdomen.

Male

In a male, testicles may not have descended but the penis is readily visible (fig. 3).

Female

In a female, there is a vulva located beneath the anus.

■ **Cat**

■ Raise the tail to reveal the external genitals, which are nearer the anus in cats than in dogs.

Male

In a male under 1 month old the testicles may not have appeared in the scrotum, and, even if they have, they are so small they may easily be confused with vulvar lips. It is therefore better to examine the shape of the genital orifice which is round in males (fig. 1 on next page).

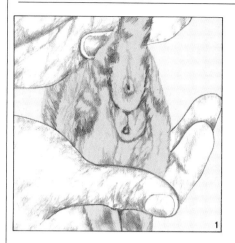
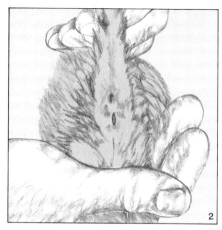

Female

In a female, the vulva looks like a vertical slit (fig. 2). Furthermore, the distance from the anus is smaller than in the male.

JUDGING THE STATE OF HEALTH

■ **Activity and appetite**

■ Even if the animal is frightened, it must be alert, with a watchful look; apathetic or depressed behaviour is often a sign of illness.
Refusal of food in animals just rescued, or collected from the breeder, may be due to fear and confusion, and need cause no worry if it does not exceed one day.

■ **Body temperature**

■ Marked variations in body temperature are a good indication of a poor state of health. See the chapter on how to measure and interpret body temperature (p. 54).

■ **State of hydration**

■ Prolonged lack of water, as well as loss of fluid through diarrhea and vomiting leads to gradual dehydration in an animal. The surest sign of adequate hydration is the normal elasticity of the skin.
In normal health, gripping a fold of skin between index finger and thumb, raising it and letting go, will result in the skin springing back to its normal position. If the animal is dehydrated, the skin feels stiff rather than elastic and the fold disappears slowly after staying in place for a few seconds (fig. 3 and 4).

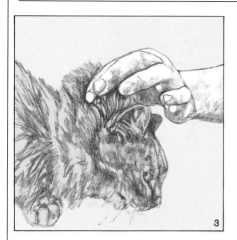

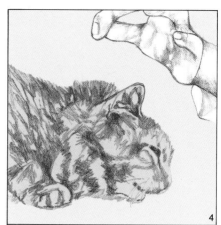

■ Eyes

Kittens:

1. male; 2 female

3.-4. Assessing a state of
hydration

5. Examining the upper part
of the white of the eye

6. How to uncover the third
eyelid

■ The eyes should always be cleaned regularly and carefully so there are no accumulated discharges such as mucus or pus, or dry crusts at the edge of the lids.

If there is a small deposit of moist or dried mucus in the inner angle of the eye, it should not be regarded as abnormal.

You can see if there is an inflamed conjunctival membrane by looking at the upper part of the white of the eye (fig. 5) or at the third eyelid. This can be protruded by carefully pressing down on the eyeball through the covering of the upper eyelid (fig. 6).

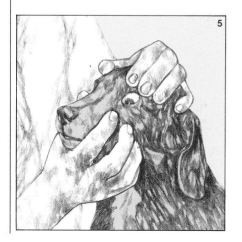

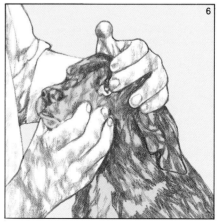

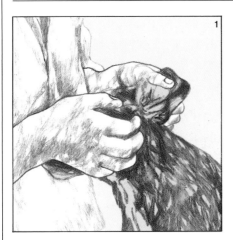

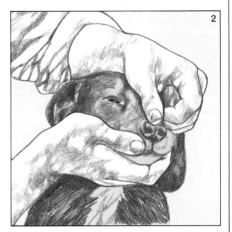

| **Ears** | ■ Check that the ears are held correctly: if there is a drooping ear which is always being scratched or shaken it may well be infected. Check the inside of the flap which should be clean and a normal flesh–pink colour, with no suggestion of inflammation (which will make it a deeper pink–red). No smell should be detectable (fig. 1). |

■ Ears

■ Check that the ears are held correctly: if there is a drooping ear which is always being scratched or shaken it may well be infected.
Check the inside of the flap which should be clean and a normal flesh–pink colour, with no suggestion of inflammation (which will make it a deeper pink–red). No smell should be detectable (fig. 1).

■ Nose

■ It is an important sign of upper respiratory tract infection if nasal discharges can be seen, or their dried residues (crusts), around the nostrils (fig. 2).

■ Anus

■ You should examine the hair surrounding the anus and the underside of the tail to check for traces of diarrhea.

■ Skin and coat

■ A healthy animal should have a thick, glossy coat but do not be alarmed if a stray looks in a bad state; its coat may merely be dirty. You should, on the other hand, examine the coat for bare patches of skin or obvious abrasions.
Check the skin by parting the hair all over from head to tail and see whether there is any evidence of parasites.

Fleas

Fleas are most easily found along the spine, especially just in front of the tail and around the neck (fig. 4). Often you will not be able to find them directly but their droppings can usually be spotted (fig. 3). These are flecks like commas or spirals,

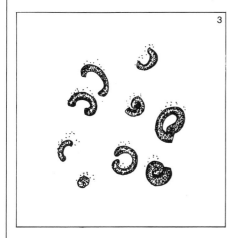

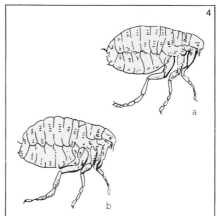

1. Examination of the ear
2. Examination of the nostrils
3. Flea droppings, enlarged
4. Fleas: a) dog flea; b) cat flea

brownish–black in colour. If you are in doubt, check the shape with a magnifying glass. Better still, you can put some on a piece of paper or cotton wool and moisten with a drop of water: if they dissolve spreading a red stain, they are flea droppings; if not, they are probably merely bits of grit or ash.

Ticks

These infect mainly dogs from early spring until autumn. They are firmly fixed to the skin, mostly on the ears and adjacent areas, the neck and between the toes of the paws. They should be easy to recognize and distinguish from cysts and pimples by the presence of four pairs of legs at the bottom (fig. 1a and 1b on the next page), although if swollen, these features are much less obvious. Frequently they are mistaken for small, darkly pigmented tumours.

Lice

These, again, are skin parasites but are less common than fleas and ticks. They are found mainly on the head of young animals. You can identify them with a magnifying glass: as they are only about 1–2 mm (½–¾ in) in length; or presume their presence on finding eggs (nits) securely attached to hairs (fig. 2a and 2b on next page).

Skin changes

The following are the most common changes to the skin that you will notice:
– Areas of reddening and spots, sometimes slightly inflamed.
– Areas of swelling with scabs making the skin moist

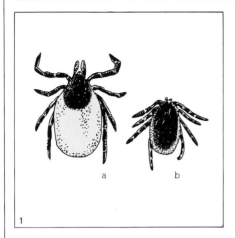

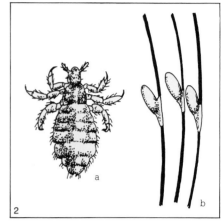

1. Ticks:
a) male; b) female
2. a) lice; b) lice eggs on hair

and sticky, at times evil smelling.
– Crusts.
– Nodules in the skin or just beneath it, of various shapes and sizes.
– Wounds of varying sizes and depth.

If you find traces of one or more of the above indications of poor health, or equally if there are signs of the following ailments, consult the vet at once:
– Sneezing, coughing, difficult breathing (possibly with wheezing, panting or other noises).
– Lameness, loss of balance or paralysis.
– Vomiting, diarrhea, constipation.
– Abnormal urination: excessive amounts in association with an increased thirst; difficult urination.

DIET

Generally the first thing to be concerned with when you find a stray is giving it the correct food and drink.

■ **Up to 1 month old**

■ In the first month of life puppies and kittens will need milk which is as similar as possible in make-up to that of their mother.
Cow's milk, although the most readily available, is very different to bitch's and cat's milk. It may cause diarrhea, but the main problem with it is that the

nutrients are over-diluted. There are many specially formulated substitute milks for puppies and kittens on sale now. If you do not have any of these, a domestic substitute can easily be made up:

– Take a glass of full cow's milk and heat it indirectly in a bowl over simmering water to about 50°C (120°F) so that it feels warm but does not scald.
– Add a spoonful of cream, a spoonful of egg yolk and a drop of lemon juice.
– Mix together all the ingredients until you have a smooth milk.

Number of feeds

If the animal's eyes are still shut, then feed it at least 6 times a day; otherwise 4 or 5 times at regular intervals throughout the day.

Quantity of milk per feed

The amount of milk per feed depends on age and size. For kittens and small dogs you should use the lower limit.
– From 10–15 ml (⅓–½ fl oz) if the umbilical cord or its remnants are still present (one tablespoon is the equivalent of about 10 ml [⅓ fl oz]).
– From 20–30 ml (¾–1 fl oz) if the puppy or kitten is well developed though its eyes and ears are still shut.
– From 30–60 ml (1–2 fl oz) if the eyes and ears are open but milk teeth are still absent.
– From 60–120 ml (2–4 fl oz) if the first teeth have started to erupt.

How to give the milk

If you do not have a proper feeding bottle, large syringes (without a needle) may be used for small animals. If the mouth is big enough, a baby's bottle may do.
Check that the milk is tepid and fill the bottle. Feed the puppy or kitten by holding it in a position as near as possible to a natural one (fig. 1 on the next page). You may find some difficulty in getting the animal to accept the bottle or substitute container the first time. However, you should be patient and persist, repeatedly wetting the mouth with milk to stimulate its suckling.
After feeding you should clean the animal as its natural mother would. Pass a finger or a bit of clean cloth moistened in tepid water gently over the

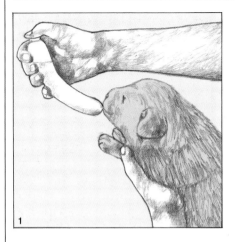 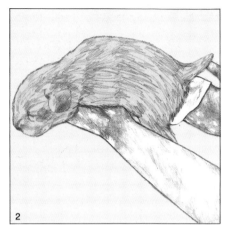

1. Feeding a newborn puppy
2. Massaging the abdomen to stimulate elimination

■ **Weaned puppies and kittens**

mouth and body in the direction of the coat; by massaging the abdomen, anus and external genitals you will promote elimination (fig. 2), after which it is best to clean and dry the animal to avoid urine and motions irritating the skin.

■ If the animal has all its first teeth and is more independent and sure in its movements, solid food must be given as well.
Until the vet gives precise instructions, confine yourself to mixing baby food or rusk-like breakfast cereal with good minced meat and adding a little tepid cow's milk or formulated substitute milk for puppies and kittens, particularly if diarrhea develops when cow's milk is given. You can also use special puppy biscuits and a vitamin/mineral supplement (following the manufacturer's recommended amounts). Other freshly cooked meats, fish and chicken can be substituted as long as they are boned thoroughly and chopped finely.
After 2 months the diet can be the same as that of adults. On the first occasion, it is best to give only boiled minced meat. Dog and cat biscuits may be indigestible for the very young or those with stomach upsets; try adding them in small amounts from the second meal, gradually increasing the amount later if the animal accepts and digests them. You can carry on until they make up about half the food.

Number of daily feeds

There should be 3 or 4 feeds per day well distributed throughout the day. Try to keep feeding to regular times every day. This is beneficial to the animal's health and will make toilet training easier.

Amount of food

The table shows how much food should be given to young kittens and puppies.

	Body weight	Quantity
Kittens	0.5 kg/1 lb	70g/2½ oz
	1 kg/2¼ lb	100g/3½ oz
	1.5 kg/3¼ lb	150g/5 oz
Puppies	0.5 kg/1 lb	70g/2½ oz
	1 kg/2¼ lb	100g/3½ oz
	2 kg/4½ lb	175g/6 oz
	3 kg/6½ lb	225g/8 oz
	4 kg/9 lb	300g/10 oz

■ **Adults**

■ If you notice the animal is very thirsty, you should give it a bowl of water. If the total requirement is large, it is better to give the liquid in several small quantities.
– Use fresh tap water and avoid milk, which it may not be able to digest. In the case of dehydration (see p. 228), you can add a teaspoonful of sugar per glass of water.
– Check the temperature of the water. It should not be cold and preferably tepid.

Avoid giving the animal food just before or just after it has drunk a large quantity of water. Allow at least 1 hour between feeding and substantial drinking. Until you have established that the animal has no digestive troubles such as vomiting or diarrhea, keep its diet simple with easily digestible foods, be they home-prepared or commercial products. Feed the animal with home-prepared cooked meat or fish, cut in pieces or minced, or tinned dog or cat food; biscuits, or any potatoes, bread and vegetables should at first be given only in small amounts and then gradually increased if accepted.

Number of feeds

Even if the animal is very hungry, do not offer too much food at once. It is far better to feed it several times a day. After two days, twice should be sufficient for a cat and once for most dogs. Food should be given at the same times each day.

General feeding guide

A dog or a cat should, as far as is possible, be fed on what it is used to. New foods will therefore have to be introduced slowly. Always make sure the food is free of fish or chicken bones and that fresh clean water is available.

Dogs needs a good proportion of high-quality protein in the form of tinned or home-cooked red meat, chicken or fish. Carbohydrate for energy will make up the rest of the food in the form of suitable biscuits, or rice, potatoes and bread. Cooked vegetables can be added although often the animal will not accept them and they are by no means essential. Vitamins and minerals are mainly obtained from tinned food and dog biscuits anyway.

A cat's diet should have a larger protein component and little carbohydrate. Feed cats twice daily on tinned cat food or home-cooked protein foods.

RECOMMENDED DAILY INTAKE

	Body weight	Quantity
Dog	5 kg / 11 lb	250g/ 9 oz
	10 kg / 22 lb	400g/14 oz
	15 kg / 33 lb	550g/ 1 lb
	20 kg / 44 lb	650g/1¼ lb
	25 kg / 55 lb	750g/1½ lb
	30 kg / 66 lb	850g/1¾ lb
Cat	2.5-3 kg / 5-7 lb	150g/ 5 oz
	4 kg / 8-9 lb	200g/ 7 oz

A general guide to quantities is 15 g per 1 kg (½ oz per 1 lb) body weight but smaller animals may need relatively more and larger ones relatively less.

When you visit the vet, you should ask about more specific diets or changes that may be required.

CLEANING

Do not bathe the animal unless you are sure that it is fit. Chilling after a bath may make disorders worse and aggravate problems with breathing, digestion or rheumatism. If necessary, clean the eyes and ears as explained on pages 46 and 48 and cleanse the dirtier areas of the skin only with a wet sponge.

When a dog is fit, and particularly if it is foul smelling, it can be bathed with a special dog shampoo, but make sure it is completely dry afterwards. While a bath is not absolutely necessary, and often difficult if the dog does not co-operate, you should groom it thoroughly with a dog brush or comb. Moulting cats will need to be combed and brushed to remove excess hair. This will avoid the cat licking loose hairs which, when ingested, form fur balls in the stomach. Also, grooming allows you to assess the animal's health from its coat and to strengthen the bond between you and the animal.

It is best to ask the advice of a vet before giving anti-parasite and worming treatments in order to be sure that it is completely necessary and that the most suitable type is used.

Birds

Unlike the cats and dogs we find, which are usually simply lost or abandoned, rescued birds are nearly always injured or in distress.

In both the town and the country, we sometimes come across birds which need help because they are sick, injured or unable to fly or feed themselves. In towns and cities pigeons, blackbirds and sparrows commonly take up residence in streets and buildings and are often the subject of accidents and illness. In the country, especially after a storm, you may find a bird's nest which has fallen from a tree on to the ground. Occasionally one comes across a bird which is injured and unable to move.

The way to pick up these birds and help them in these situations is described in the chapter on approaching, catching and transporting wild animals on page 239. This section gives some advice on helping the little creatures to recover.

REARING NESTLINGS

If you find a nest of young birds that has fallen on to the ground in a storm, or if your canary or budgerigar abandons its young, you can act in place of the parents and feed the nestlings artificially.
First of all, put the nest in a box with a lid which can be kept closed. In the dark the birds will be quiet and not try to escape. As you lift the lid to open the box, the birds will open their beaks to ask for food.
There are special products on sale for the artificial feeding of birds. If you cannot obtain any of these, you can prepare a paste consisting of hard-boiled egg yolk and broken biscuit crumbs moistened with water and mixed to a creamy texture. The food is then offered to the birds on the end of a stick.

FEEDING ADULT BIRDS

Canaries are graniverous birds. They will eat a seed mix of white seed, broken oats, millet varieties, rape and cole seed, niger seed and sesame seed. You can supplement the diet with fruit and vegetables such as apples, carrots and greenstuff.
A budgerigar's, lovebird's or small parrakeet's diet is, again, mainly graniverous. They should be given a mix of millet (Japanese, plate, red or white millets), white seed and whole or hulled oats. To this, add vegetables such as cabbage, watercress, lettuce and stalks from green and red peppers.
The large group of attractive, small cage-birds including waxbills, Java sparrows, Zebra finches and Moluccan Mannikins all share a similar diet and should be given an assortment of Senegal setaria, panicum and white pearl millet, white seed, mulled oats, sesame, poppy or niger seed. They will rarely accept fruit and vegetables.
The three main species of cage-talking parrots, the African Grey Parrot, the You-you and the South American predominantly green species, *Amazona amazonica* will need a more varied diet since they are omnivorous.
The Minah bird is shiny black with two lateral yellow caruncles. It is an insectivorous bird and needs a feed for insect-eating birds, plus fruit and greenstuff.
You can obtain all these various bird-food mixes from pet shops.

APPROACHING, CATCHING AND TRANSPORTING A WILD ANIMAL

The first-aid measures to be taken with wild animals in an emergency situation are generally the same as those described for domestic animals, except that the first aider will run more risk of being hurt and will have to pay more care and attention. It is, therefore, even more necessary to ensure the intervention of the vet as soon as possible.

■ **Respect for wildlife**

Approaching a wild animal entails imposing our presence on an animal which is not used to having human beings around and will flee from them in normal circumstances.

It is very important to bear this in mind if you want to help out a wild animal in trouble without aggravating the situation in any way.

Wild animals have the innate ability to survive and ensure the perpetuation of the species within their own habitat, fighting off any predators, including man, and natural competitors. This survival instinct in some species is irrevocable: a wounded sparrow or swallow will not tolerate being caught and handled, while other animals will accept help more easily and lose their instinct for freedom more readily.

■ Man will instinctively try to tame animals and subordinate them to his own needs. This interference with nature can cause serious damage to the lives of wild animals, which of necessity fear man and his dog or cat.

A few days of captivity, the time taken to recover from a wound, may be enough for an eagle or falcon wrongly handled to develop abnormal habits and lose forever the ability to find their own food. In other words, even if we can help an animal regain its health and vitality, releasing it back into the wild may be very difficult or even impossible. This is especially true for predators (eagles, kites, wolves etc.), in which the maintaining of active, good health and the presence of a strong predatory instinct are essential for survival.

It is, therefore, necessary to bear in mind that you will be able to help some wild animals by capturing them and aiding their recovery, but not with the aim of releasing them afterwards.

■ **Likelihood of survival**

■ Another consideration, when assessing the degree of first aid to give the wild animal, is that an animal which does not resist capture by trying to flee, or that does not act aggressively if it cannot escape, must be very weak. It therefore may well not survive handling and transportation and a period of captivity. It would be better in this case to leave the animal to its natural fate and think of the creature simply as a link in the long food chain which runs from grass and tiny insects to the ultimate predator, man.

However, it is often hard to resist a spontaneous gesture of help, which is basically a noble one, especially if the sight of the animal arouses feelings of pity and affection.

■ **Dangers in giving first aid**

■ Many animals, even if they look small and delicate, can be dangerous, either because they are aggressive or because they carry diseases that can affect man.

PRECAUTIONS

Before approaching a wild animal that has been injured or fallen into a trap, assess the risks that you may be running in order to rescue it.

They could be of two types:
– potential aggression with bites and scratches;
– potential diseases transmitted by contact.

■ **Transmission of diseases**

■ An animal that attacks and inflicts injury, and which may in fact be dying, can transmit various infections, some of which can be very dangerous, and even fatal, to man.

In the table on the following page, we list some important examples of diseases carried by wild animals, their specific carriers and the modes of transmission.

Disease	Carrier	Transmission
Rabies Viral disease which causes nervous disorders *Always fatal in man*	Red fox, feral cat, polecat, all carniverous predators	Bites, deep wounds and scratches
Tularemia Acute or cardiac bacterial disease *Sometimes fatal in man*	Hare, wild rabbit, squirrel, pheasant, partridge, quail etc.	By contact through abrasions and cuts in the skin
Tuberculosis Serious bacterial disease with a slow course and difficult recovery *Sometimes fatal in man*	Mammals, birds, primates, reptiles	By contact and inhalation
Leptospirosis Acute, cardiac or septicemic bacterial disease *Sometimes fatal in man*	Mice, rats, guinea pigs	By direct contact, through small cuts in the skin and by ingestion
Sarcoptic Mange A parasitic dermatitis	Carnivores (fox, dogs)	By contact
Tick Fever Course similar to influenza *Rarely fatal*	Pigeons	Bites from ticks on birds

■ **Aggressive reactions**	■ While keeping your distance, you should try to establish exactly what type of animal is involved and what injured state it might be in.
Species	It is useful to know what species the animal belongs to and whether it is a predator or not. As a result, you will have an idea how aggressive it will be in its reaction to you.
Condition	Observe the physical condition of the animal and how alert it is.

| Aggression | The level of aggression will depend on the species and the gravity of the situation. Generally a predator is more dangerous than a non-predator; an animal caught in a snare can react violently even if seriously wounded which may result in severe injury to anyone trying to help it and worsen the condition of the animal.
It is best to be wary of unusual behaviour (especially in wolves or cats and dogs living in the wild), for example one that does not try to run away but comes towards humans. This precaution is vital in areas where rabies is rife since a lack of normal fear is an early feature of rabies.
Before touching a wild animal it is a good idea to use a stick to test from a distance how fiercely it reacts. |

RISKS IN HANDLING

When we approach a wild animal, it will interpret how we behave and the way we observe it as if we were predators. This naturally arouses fear, panic and desperate attempts to escape. It is therefore best to approach sideways, looking at the animal as little as possible and recognizing the way it will probably defend itself before taking hold of it.

■ **Birds**	■ Birds have various ways of attacking and defending themselves.
Beaks	They can use the beak, which is surprisingly strong and hard, aided by the neck which stretches considerably. Many species use their beak for defense, while others (birds of prey), though opening it to threaten, rarely bite.
Claws	The claws are the main tool used by birds of prey and are very dangerous because they are pointed and curved: they cause extensive injury and it is difficult to break free from them. Many birds of prey, if unable to flee, pretend to be dead, remaining immobile with an open beak. Beware of this.
Wing beats	Wing beats are typically used by big water birds and by predators to keep an enemy at bay. This is not dangerous if you take care.

■ Mammals

■ Methods of defense and attack used by mammals are different but no less effective.

Teeth

The bite of many species can cause severe wounds and transmit infections. Take great care with small mammals (hare, squirrel, dormouse, polecat, marmot, marten etc.) and carnivorous predators in general (fox, wild cat etc.). Protect your hands with a strong cloth or leather gloves, and always disinfect injuries at once.

Claws

Many species, other than carnivorous predators, may look tame but can inflict severe injury and extensive scratches with their claws (squirrel, badger, hare etc.).

Horns

Horns are the typical weapons of defense and attack in wild ruminants (stag, roebuck, chamois etc.).

Spines

An armature of spines provides the hedgehog with its vicious defense. To handle them, thick leather gloves are essential, or else you will have to devise special tactics.

CAPTURE AND HANDLING

When you are going to capture and handle a wild animal, you should always bear certain things in mind. If you take the wrong decision or make a wrong move, you could do more harm than good.

– Never be too hasty deciding to capture and take a wild animal home, above all with nestlings which are often best left where they are found. Leave them sheltered from predators so that the parents can soon find them again.
– Keep as calm as possible while you are catching and handling wild animals, avoiding sudden movements and noise.
– Touch the animal as little as possible; do not bother trying to befriend the animal by stroking it. If it is wild, even if sick, it will not easily accept your presence.
– Keep the animal for the minimum amount of time needed to cure it, and then release it. This is the kindest way to treat animals.

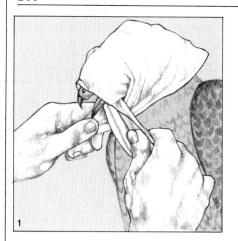

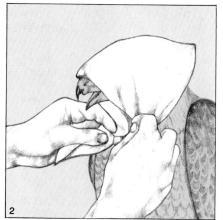

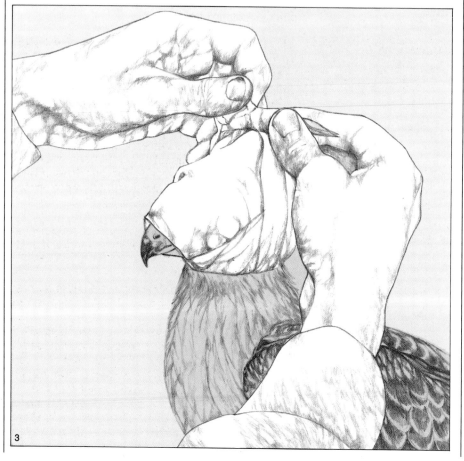

1.-2.-3. Stages in putting a
hood on a raptor
4. How the claws of a raptor
are tied

– Always hold birds low down, i.e. near your waist, and far away from your face and eyes.
– Protect your hands with gloves and promptly disinfect any wounds, bearing in mind you may need an anti-tetanus injection.

In most cases when meeting an injured animal, no useful equipment for capturing is to hand. You will have to use improvised methods to restrain the wild animal but try to ensure minimum upset and injury to the animal from handling.

Birds and mammals

■ **Birds**

■ The best way to approach a bird is sideways without looking straight at it.

Large birds

One way to capture a large bird is to throw a blanket over it to prevent it escaping. A small amount of pressure on this covering will immobilize the animal. Then slowly lift the blanket and securely grasp the bird just behind the head; with the other hand restrain the wings, and keep them from beating. If possible, blindfold the bird with a handkerchief but take care not to hurt its eyes or obstruct the nostrils (fig. 1, 2 and 3): an animal that cannot see will move less and is less frightened. If the bird tries to bite, fasten its beak with a rubber band or a piece of tape (take care not to cover the nostrils).

Small birds

For small birds the covering must not be too heavy: it is better to use a towel or pullover, applying it with great care.

Raptors

Raptors (eagle, falcon, kite etc.) can cause a great deal of harm and a degree of skill is needed in handling them.
If the animal remains still and lets itself be handled (remember a bird of prey's trick of feigning death), first the head and eyes should be covered and then the claws secured. Often, however, the animal reacts and capture becomes difficult; a fairly heavy blanket may be used to restrain the bird. So long as it is in the dark, it will not try to fight back. From under the blanket, the claws are then located and uncovered with the animal seeing as little as

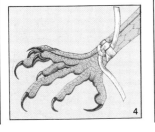

possible. Once the claws are made safe (by a secure grip or with a flat piece of tape to bind them together, [fig. 4 on previous page]), the animal can be uncovered, provided the wings are kept close to the body.

■ Mammals

■ There are different guidelines for the various species according to the size and build of the animal.

Small mammals

Small mammals are often hard to catch, being quick and liable to bite. Those with a long tail (squirrel, dormouse etc.) must be seized by the tail and kept

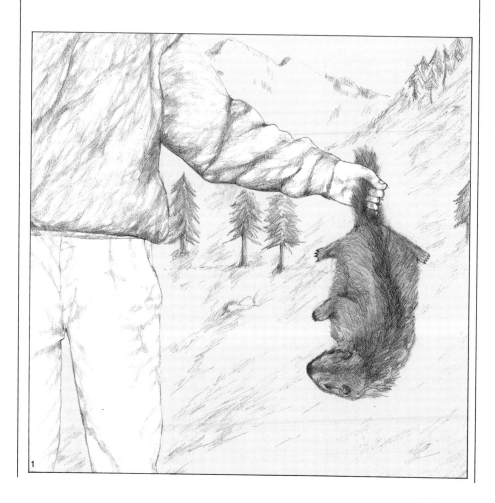

1

well away from your body (fig. 1); those with a short tail (field mouse, guinea pig, hamster, mole etc.) and Mustelidae such as weasels, skunks and badgers must be held firmly just behind the head, by the loose skin of the neck, but wear gloves of thick leather or cloth.

Mustelidae

1. How to grasp a small mammal by the tail
2. Catching a fox with a dog catcher

Mustelidae (polecat, weasel, ermine, etc.) are vicious, dangerous and hard to approach if not in a weakened state. It is best to use a strong net or a blanket to immobilize the animal. As soon as it is captured, put the animal into a suitable container for transportation. Squirrels need the same treatment.

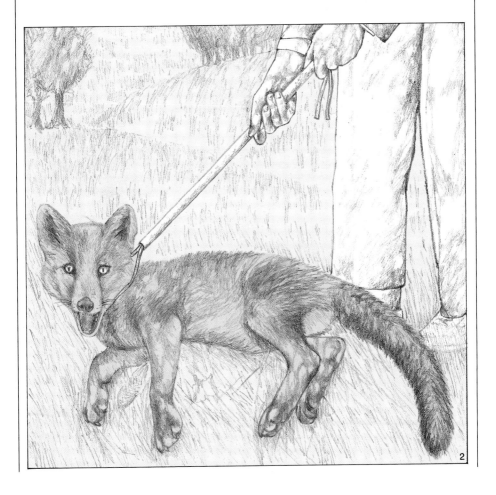

Hares and wild rabbits

Hares and wild rabbits must be held by both ears (never by just one alone) and by the skin of the back at the same time, while paying attention to the position of the feet which can inflict painful scratches. Do not be distracted by the piercing cries of the animal during both its capture and subsequent handling.

Hedgehog

To catch a hedgehog you need either thick fur or leather gloves, or you must again restrain the animal within a blanket or a newspaper, lifting the whole arrangement without ever touching the animal itself.

Fox or badger

Faced with a fox or badger, you should be very careful: in many cases you may have to resort to using a dog catcher. This could even be assembled on the spot using bits and pieces that are to hand (fig. 2 on the previous page).

TRANSPORTATION

It is important to choose an appropriate container to transport the animal in.

For large non-predatory birds, especially water birds (swan, goose etc.), it is often enough to wrap the animal in a blanket or newspaper, or confine it in a bag of sacking with one corner removed to allow its head and neck to stick out (fig. 1). You could also use cloth or soft leather bags with a zip which are especially good for carrying long-tailed birds (pheasant, peacock etc.). You can put their body inside and head and tail outside (fig. 1 on p. 250).

For small birds, cardboard boxes with little holes to allow breathing are ideal containers: the animal can be left free inside and, ideally, it should be blindfolded with a handkerchief to lessen any violent struggle to get out.

Raptors can be carried in large cardboard boxes, either closed but ventilated by small holes, or open, with the head covered by a handkerchief, two ends of which are tied around the beak (fig. 2 on p. 250). Never use the wickerwork or metal wire baskets used for carrying cats: they can cause serious injuries to large birds (e.g. raptors and others).

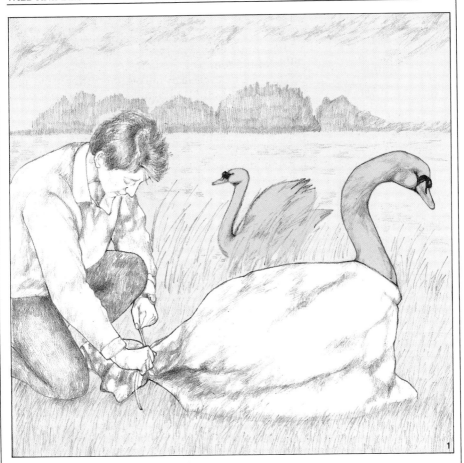

1. Preparing a swan for transportation

Small mammals can be carried in perforated cardboard boxes only for very short trips as, with time, they will eat through the cardboard and escape. Therefore it is better to use perforated wooden or metal boxes (like biscuit tins). For long trips, wicker baskets can be used for hares, wild rabbits etc., if they are large enough and covered with a cloth to make the inside dark.

Metal cages intended for birds may be used for the more dangerous animals (squirrels, Mustelidae), but they must be covered with a cloth that will keep the inside dark but let air in.

An injured animal always likes shelter and darkness

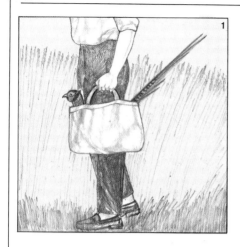 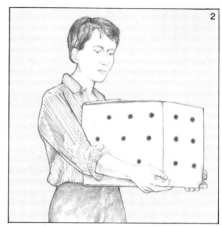

Transportation of an animal:
1. Medium-sized bird
2. Raptor

and this also avoids struggling and attempts at escape. Leave the animal free inside the darkened container to allow it to adopt a natural posture during transportation. For big mammals (fox, badger) it would be preferable to use a wooden chest which is strong and suitably ventilated.

Having arrived at your destination and whilst waiting for the intervention of the vet, you should carry out the following steps to ensure the maximum comfort and safety for the animal:

– Put the animal in a quiet, dark and warm spot, but away from direct heat sources. Ideal temperatures are 22–25°C (70–77°F) for adults, 25–30°C (77–86°F) for any young or newly born animal.
– Make a bed with rags or newspaper (not straw or hay unless it is for hares, rabbits and large wild herbivores).
– Put water (perhaps slightly sugared) within reach but do not force food on the animal. It is unlikely to eat for some days after an injury.
– Leave all parts of the body free to move including the beak.
– Small animals should be put in suitably large and well ventilated boxes, with a warm hot-water bottle in one corner of the container. Aim at a temperature of 25°C (77°F).
– Areas and objects that have been in contact with the animal must be carefully disinfected afterwards.

PROTECTION OF WILD ANIMALS

When catching a wild animal, remember there are specific laws for their protection. It is also important to bear in mind that these will differ from one country to another. Some species are considered game and can be hunted only at certain times of the year and others are protected (sometimes being the subject of special legislation). You should therefore take care when considering giving first aid to a wild animal since in many countries it is a crime to catch a protected species, or game out of season. This is another reason why a wild animal should be caught and kept only after serious consideration, and on finding one, it should be reported to the proper authority. After that you might consider transferring it to a special sanctuary for wild animals, if you locate one, or approach an association for the protection of animals of that species.